# Weight Loss Boss

# Weight Loss Boss

## How to finally **win at losing**— and take charge in an **out-of-control food world**

### David Kirchhoff
President and CEO, Weight Watchers International, Inc.

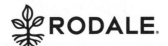

© 2012 Weight Watchers International, Inc.

Rodale books may be purchased for business or promotional use or for special sales. For information, please write to: Special Markets Department, Rodale Inc., 733 Third Avenue, New York, NY 10017.

Printed in the United States of America
Rodale Inc. makes every effort to use acid-free ♾, recycled paper ♻.

Book design by Elizabeth Neal,
with George Karabotsos
Illustrations by Scott Menchin

Cover photography by Matt Jones; styling by Mindy Saad
Grooming by Anja Grassegger using Dior Homme at Factory Downtown
Food styling by Matt Vohr and prop styling by Rebecca Donnelly

Page 26: Graph reprinted from *The Lancet*, "The Global Obesity Pandemic: Shaped by Global Drivers and Local Environments"; Vol. 378/9793; Boyd A. Swinburn, Gary Sacks, Kevin D. Hall, Klim McPherson, Diane T. Finegood, Marjory L. Moodie, Steven L. Gortmaker; pages 804–814; ©2011; with permission from Elsevier.

Page 36: From *I Got This: How I Changed My Ways and Lost What Weighed Me Down* by Jennifer Hudson, copyright ©2012 by Jennifer Hudson. Used by permission of Dutton, a division of Penguin Group (USA) Inc.

Page 85: MyPlate graphics reprinted courtesy of the USDA Center for Nutrition Policy and Promotion (CNPP)

Page 110: Fogg Behavior Model printed with permission from B. J. Fogg

Library of Congress Cataloging-in-Publication Data is on file with the publisher.

ISBN-13: 978-1-60961-901-5 hardcover

Distributed to the trade by Macmillan

2   4   6   8   10   9   7   5   3   1   hardcover

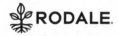

**RODALE.**

We inspire and enable people to improve their lives and the world around them.
www.rodalebooks.com

To every Weight Watchers leader, receptionist,
clerk, and coach, past, present, and future.
Keep the fires burning!

# Contents

INTRODUCTION:
## Staying Healthy in an Unhealthy World ....................... 1
Obesity is the great tectonic plate moving across the dinner table
toward you and me—crushing our health (and our national economy).
Defeat isn't inevitable! Here, my five rules for taking off—and
keeping off—the weight for life.

---

**PART I**    FROM THIN TO HEAVY AND BACK AGAIN: A WEIGHT LOSS ODYSSEY

---

CHAPTER 1:
## Paging Dr. Freud—Early Influences and Food Attitudes ................................................................................. 21
A look back at my too skinny youth, how genetics affect everything
from fat distribution to cravings, and how yesterday's habits and sneaky
behaviors affect how I lose it around food today.

**WEIGHT WATCHERS PROFILE:** Jennifer Hudson     36
"When I sing 'Feeling Good,' that's for real!"

CHAPTER 2:
## Letting Loose in an Obesogenic Environment ....... 39
How a sudden change of environment (and the foods that pollute it)
can bring on weight gain of epic proportions.

**WEIGHT WATCHERS PROFILE:** Derrick Deaton     48
"You can do this! I know you can!"

**PART II**

# BE THE BOSS OF YOUR OWN WEIGHT LOSS: FOOD, TOOLS, AND STRATEGIES TO TAKE CHARGE FOR LIFE

# Foreword

I love this book. My passion for it isn't sparked by the fact that it is penned by one of my heroes, although David *is* a heroic character. It isn't because it is about his journey to wellness, though I respect his journey. Nor is it because this book is written by a guy wittingly talking about weight loss, while so few men really know or understand the subject and even fewer talk about it. And just because David is the CEO of the most successful weight loss company in America wouldn't make me fall in love with his writing. While those are key reasons why this book is important and informative, they don't explain my passion any more than I love my wife because she is a safe driver.

Before I explain any further, though, let's consider why still another book about weight loss is needed, and maybe why only David can write it this powerfully.

First: David asserts that obesity is a bi-gender issue. His personal success story of trying to get back to a healthy frame confirms that men can retake their health as well as women can. He doesn't just talk the talk, he lives it.

Second, he argues that weight loss is no longer just *your* decision: Whether the United States will compete for jobs and keep its freedoms—or conversely need to ration medical care—will depend on whether you control your weight. Increased girth brings hikes in costly chronic diseases such as hypertension, type 2 diabetes, inflammation, and their consequences—arthritis, heart disease and stroke, and cancer. These diseases are making us less competitive for jobs and are breaking budgets as well. And most important, unlike many other authors, David understands that maintenance may be the most important phase of weight loss—the fact that he shows us how to pull it off makes this book unique.

But the real reason I'm crazy about this book is that David, with all his personal experience, confirms some of the conclusions I've formed from coaching just a fraction of the people he and his company try to help daily: that you need to change your environment and attitude while making your food choices and activity habits automatic. The food gods are too powerful for mere mortal willpower to win the battle with ice cream. For anyone experienced in coaching others on how to gain their ideal weight and waist (not a Barbie or Ken waist), you have to love what David does in this book.

He tells you that getting to your lifetime weight goal is about making yourself and your health a priority and explains how you can do so. He tells you the reason for establishing habits such as eating the same healthy breakfast and lunch every day and explains how you can do so. He tells you about the importance of changing your environment and explains how you can do so. He tells you about transforming enough bad habits into good habits to establish a healthy lifestyle to last forever and explains how you can do so. He uses the vast experience of Weight Watchers patrons to infuse the story with real data and journeys other than his own. Yet what really makes me love this book is that David is man (or woman) enough to be humble and honest about his and others' struggles to lose excess weight and then to maintain an ideal waist, as well as candid about how difficult that process is. May you be savvy enough to be like David and change your environment so you can make only smart decisions, and lucky enough to absorb his wisdom and have the waist you want. May you enjoy—and be—a *Weight Loss Boss.*

**—MICHAEL F. ROIZEN, MD,**
chief wellness officer, and J Gorman and Family chair
of the Wellness Institute, Cleveland Clinic

# Acknowledgments

This book was born out of a simple suggestion in early 2009 that I think about writing a blog. An old college friend of mine, Dan Abrams—of TV news fame—was trying to give me some pointers about different ways of creating a bigger profile for the Weight Watchers name. The idea of a blog stuck with me, but I had no idea what to write about. Then it occurred to me that very few men talk or write about their experience with weight loss. I made the decision to start reflecting on my personal experience with my own weight rather than as the CEO of Weight Watchers. I named the blog Man Meets Scale, and so began a 3-year experiment.

This book draws heavily from the blog and includes many of my favorite passages. Therefore, my first thanks have to go to anyone who helped me with the blog, including my colleagues in editorial (Nancy Gagliardi and Theresa Di Masi), marketing (Lee Hurley), as well as our Web design team (led by Adam Cricchio) who helped make it look a little less amateurish.

Suffice to say, I could not have written this book without actually losing weight. For this, I thank the so many amazing, passionate, brilliant, and wonderful people who run our Weight Watchers meetings. I have never been in one of your meetings when I didn't learn something new, even if I didn't speak the language. I not only learned from our leaders and receptionists, but I also learned much from my fellow Weight Watchers members. I am honored to be one of your peeps. Most important, to my two primary meetings leaders: thanks to Michael Filan for giving me my first Weight Watchers tutorial, and special thanks to Liz Josefsberg who got me to goal weight and Lifetime Membership.

To this day, I'm a little shocked that my legal department ever let me go down this goofy path of oversharing personal details while still being the CEO of a publicly traded company. In particular, Terri Frank has kindly and diligently looked out for me to make sure I didn't do anything too unbelievably dumb while still letting me have lots of creative rope (just not enough to hang myself). Of course, I therefore must also thank my old friend and general counsel Jeff Fiarman for all of the above kindnesses.

Many of my views and perspectives have been heavily influenced by a lot of different people, especially my colleagues on the management team. Past and present, they include great friends and collaborators Meredith Shepherd, Mike Basone, Dave Burwick, Mel Stubbing, Ann Sardini, and my ever-indulgent-to-my-navel-gazing-exercises head of North American marketing Cheryl Callan. However, this list cannot begin to cover the influence that so many of my colleagues at Weight Watchers have had on me. So to all of you, THANK YOU! I know of no other group of people quite like the folks who work at this passionate, mission driven organization.

When I first joined Weight Watchers, I would have been cold and alone were it not for all of my early, early co-workers at the startup known as WeightWatchers.com, Inc. Standouts include Katy Huber, Sabrina LeBlanc, and Leslie Fink. However, it was my old friend and partner-in-crime Thilo Semmelbauer who probably had the greatest influence on me in the 10 years that followed, in more ways than I can count.

When I joined WeightWatchers.com, Inc., I was but a midthirties man-child with responsibility disproportionate to my experience. It may not be in fashion these days to heap praise on private equity guys, but I have to make an exception here. The good people at Invus raised me from a pup. They patiently mentored me and withstood my youthful expressions more times than I can count. Most important, they gave me and our team the support to make decisions for the long term of Weight Watchers, not just for the next quarter. So to Chris Sobecki, Jonas Fajgenbaum, Aflalo Guimaraes, and Sacha Lainovic, I offer a huge thanks for the years of insight and patience. To my mentor Philippe Amouyal, I say thank you for the endless wisdom and counsel. To my boss, Ray

Debbane, the chairman of Weight Watchers, thanks for taking a chance on a young bull-in-the-china-shop guy and helping him turn into a much better leader and executive (I hope!).

In first writing a blog about Weight Watchers and then a book, my audience should take some comfort knowing that I have some vague notion of what I'm actually talking about. They should take great comfort knowing that the chief science officer of Weight Watchers, Karen Miller-Kovach, has been looking out for me (and them) by keeping me on the straight and narrow of accepted science. For more than 12 years, Karen has been my expert, my advisor, my colleague, and my friend. I could never have achieved any of the insights in this book without her. And, of course, I am utterly indebted to my assistant Gwen Vinocur, without whom all my wheels would have fallen off.

Beyond the influences of Weight Watchers, I am indebted to the many brilliant and inspiring people who think about the topic of weight and/or behavior change each and every day. Notable influences and friends include Brian Wansink, B.J. Fogg, Richard Thaler, David Katz, Pat O'Brien, Rena Wing, George Loewenstein, Eric Finkelstein, Barbara Rolls, Dean Ornish, and many, many others. Particular thanks to Dr. Mike Roizen for always fighting the good fight to promote a healthier and more vibrant world.

So where exactly did this goofy idea for me to write a book come from? Well, none other than Dave Zinczenko, from Rodale, who sent me an e-mail suggesting that very thing. Dave then proceeded to torture me with completely ridiculous deadlines, with little regard for the fact that I actually had a day job. I suspect he found it amusing to see exactly how high he could make me jump. Nonetheless, being asked to write the book was an incredible compliment, and being supported throughout the process was an even bigger kindness.

One of Dave's biggest kindnesses was giving me a ridiculously talented team of people at Rodale to convert, trim, and sharpen my loquacious babbling into something somewhat coherent. It started with Alex Postman, who shares my naïve and passionate view of a better world of health, and then Peter Moore, editor of *Men's Health*. Somehow Peter found time when he wasn't knocking out issues of the magazine to take all of my junk and turn it into something pretty. His fingerprints are all over this book, and it's a much better and more useful document for it. Thanks, too, to Steve Perrine, whom I finally had to trust that he knows what he's doing in putting out a book, and put my faith and confidence in him. Good choice! Finally I'm grateful for the hardworking Rodale design and production teams, including George Karabotsos, Elizabeth Neal, and Nancy Bailey. On the Weight Watchers side, many thanks to Stacy Gordon for helping me navigate this whole crazy book world.

The book would not be a book if I never existed. So, of course, I have to thank my parents, Ann and Bill, on multiple levels. First thank you for making me. Thank you for feeding me. Thank you for putting me through college. Most important, thank you for sharing your curiosity, sense of humor, and your passion. For better or worse, I am who I am because of you. It's all the more horrible, then, that I pick on you in the early chapters. Sorry!!!!! To my siblings, Dan, Jenny, and Meg, thank you for not taking out a contract on me for picking on Mom and Dad in a published book. Meg, you can definitely have the illustrations if I ever write another book!

Finally, to my family. My first visit to the doctor informing me of my weight condition happened right after the birth of my first daughter, Harley. My start with Weight Watchers coincided with the birth of my second daughter, Lila. You two are the lights of my life. *Finally* finally, infinite thanks to my insanely understanding and kind wife, Sandee. Every time I wrote a new blog post, I would demand that she drop whatever she was doing, read the post, and then say "Good boy, Dave!" How can I not thank her for putting up with all of my OCD and holier-than-thou food/exercise obsessions, particularly when I first reached my goal weight. Many of my ideas for my writing came from Saturday morning coffees with Sandee. Thank you for being my muse.

# {INTRODUCTION}
# Staying Healthy in an Unhealthy World

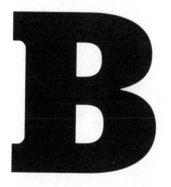EFORE I GET STARTED, there are a few important facts to know about me.

**One:** I am, in fact, the CEO of Weight Watchers, but I am also a member. I lost my weight and have maintained my loss as a member of the Weight Watchers program. In a joke that I have used too many times, I am an awful lot like the guy from the Hair Club for Men (Sy Sperling, for those with long memories). I am an unquestioning fan of my own organization for a host of reasons, not the least of which is that it helped change my life in a fundamental way. That said, this book is not primarily intended for Weight Watchers members, since much of what I've written applies to everyone who wants to lose weight.

**Two:** I am far from being the perfect role model. It took me nearly a decade to reach my goal weight, which I have now maintained for 3 years. I have a long history of failures, inadequacies, and bad habits, even today. I would tell you to do as I say, not as I do, but even my verbal commands can be suspect. Please do use your own common sense and judgment and figure out what works best for you!

**Three:** I often wish that I could go back to the year 2000, equipped with everything I know now. I came to understand more about dealing with my weight during the past 3 years of maintaining my loss than I did in 9 years of losing weight. The reason: I incorporated healthy habits into my life, which has been the key to both losing weight and keeping it off.

In my view, too many books have been written about the first 3 months of weight loss, and not nearly enough has been written about making changes that will improve how you live every day for the rest of your life. I hope to do my own part to try to change that. I have always wanted the opportunity to share the hard-earned lessons I've learned with people who are looking for a new start.

This book is my way of doing exactly that.

# Introducing
# David Kirchhoff
(Dave, to Friends)

As a kid, I was embarrassed about how skinny I was.

As an adult, I hated being fat.

Some people are never satisfied!

These days, I am pretty content with the state of my weight—203 pounds, about 40 pounds less than my peak just over a decade ago. And yet, I'm hardly on autopilot. I know that staying here will not happen by accident. I will have to keep working to make these changes permanent.

Yes, losing weight is hard, sometimes. Yes, you'll fail occasionally; I wrote the book on that (this one). But we'll also enjoy our successes—and believe me, they are achievable. While this is work, it's a job that has a big payday: It can help you live better, longer, more happily. As a special bonus, you can also look good doing it. (Style points count, right? Right!)

When I was a teenager, the very concept of being overweight was completely beyond my comprehension. In my
family, I was a bit of a genetic freak. My father is 5 foot 10, as
is my older brother, and my mother and two sisters clock in
at 5 foot 2. I shot past them (to 6 foot 3) at a blazing clip;
unfortunately, it left me looking like an underfed giraffe.
I was all arms and legs, and no matter how hard I tried, I simply couldn't gain weight. (Oh, I figured that one out big-time
later on, though.) Throughout high school, I weighed a steady
170 pounds, which made me look like I was built out of coat
hangers. There is nothing particularly cool about being able
to see all of your ribs and discern a heartbeat between them.

Then I went to college, and everything changed: I gained
45 pounds in one year. That's a disaster for most people, but
for me, I finally looked seminormal for the first time. So I
started to work out, got stronger, and rounded out my muscu-
lature. But after college, I went on to do graduate work in fat-
ness. I was steadily gaining weight from newly acquired habits
of nutritional debauchery and general slothfulness, sacrifices
I told myself I was making for a high-paced professional life.

On July 23, 1999, at the age of 32, I got my first physical in
about 7 years. In the time that elapsed between arriving in
the waiting room and getting my blood work back a week later,
my life would change.

My first shock was stepping onto my doctor's scale. Watching the nurse slide weight after weight to the right before
finally landing on 242 pounds was a punch to my expanding
gut. How did this happen? As a tall guy, I could carry my baggage pretty well, and I'd almost convinced myself that I didn't
weigh all that much. Yet, if I was being honest, I also knew that
every trip to the shower led to the recognition that I could
pinch far more than an inch. I was grabbing slabs of fat.

There was more bad news to come, with the results of my
blood work. My LDL cholesterol was at 181, and my triglycerides had spiked to 146. My doctor sat me down and told me
that both numbers were far outside of the healthy range for a

normal 32-year-old. She recommended that I start on statins but also that I get my lifestyle to a better place. She saved the worst for last: She looked me in the eye and told me that, with a body mass index (BMI) of 30, I was clinically obese.

The experience did motivate change, of a sort. I counted calories for a few weeks but soon gave up. I corrected a few obvious bad habits but not nearly enough of them. Over the next 18 months, I lost 5 to 10 pounds.

But fate delivered me to the people, and program, that would ultimately save me. Or, I should say, helped me save myself. In late December 1999, I got a job helping Weight Watchers start up its Internet business. In taking the job,

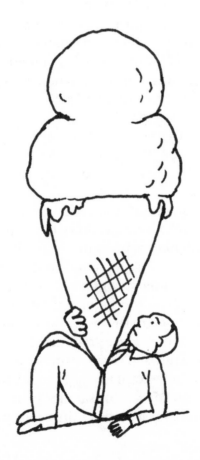

I thought it would be a nice perk to maybe lose that weight in the process. Nine years later—yes, that's right: 9 years!—I reached my goal weight, and I've been there for the last 3 years. I'll have a lot more to say about how I managed that and why it took me so long. (I have total faith that you'll be able to reach your destination faster; consider me a worst-case scenario—everybody else certainly does!) Today, my blood pressure is normal, my LDL has dropped to 76, and my triglycerides are at 82. I went from a human caution sign to green lights all around. As far as my blood numbers are concerned, I am now completely healthy.

But does that mean I am "cured"? Is the old, plush David only a memory, a ghost of Christmas cookies past?

No.

Consider my ice cream problem.

The second I pull the lid off a carton—yes, it still happens—and wield my spoon-weapon, I go all fuzzy in the head. My pulse jumps up to 140-plus, and I completely lose myself. It starts innocently enough with a single layer removal. If it's my favorite (cookie dough), I simply have to dig around for big golf balls of the frozen goo. Being slightly OCD, I then evenly eat around the hole I just made. Then I take another layer out. Soon, half of a container is gone.

I really cannot think of a single other food that has the same kind of narcotic effect on me. I'm getting excited even writing about it. For the life of me, I cannot explain why I feel this way.It almost seems animalistic when my ice cream frenzies happen; they have a powerful emotional hold over me that I will never understand.

So how do I handle it? I make sure that we do not have big containers of the stuff in the house. If I do have ice cream, it is almost always in the form of a Weight Watchers prepackaged ice-cream treat. One of the most elementary tips for binge eaters: Never, ever eat straight from the carton. As you'll see later on in the book, the key to portion control is doling out your servings, then putting away the bag, box, carton, or jug.

That's why a single serving bar is great: one and done. Except I often find myself having two.

That's why I now treat ice cream a little bit the way ex-smokers treat cigarettes: with close to zero tolerance. Generally I don't endorse banning entire categories of food, but sometimes desperate measures are required.

Because of examples like that one, I know I will always struggle with my weight. I will always have to be careful. Living healthy takes effort. It requires an education. It requires change and committing to changes so completely that they become the new normal. It is not easy, like swallowing a pill, but it is very possible. And the important thing is: I now know that the way I used to live and eat was impossible and not sustainable. And when you look at change in that light, it isn't a burden, it's a release.

As my interest in weight loss grew, I fished around on the Internet and noticed a lot of smart women launching blogs, Web sites, and Twitter feeds on my new favorite topic. Yet, for whatever reason, there were very few men doing it. For women, talking about weight and weight loss seems as natural as breathing. Guys prefer to talk about how hard that 300-pound tackle hit the running back, not what the lineman's strategy should be for achieving a 32-inch waistline. But guys need to be thinking about this stuff, too. That's a big reason why I started my blog, ManMeetsScale.blogspot.com. (I devote a whole chapter to the man versus scale problem later on.)

When I started writing the blog, I assumed that the primary audience would be men. A bunch of guys do follow the blog, but I found that many more women were checking it out and sharing their own experiences. It seemed that my challenges with weight, both how I gained it and how I struggle to keep it off, were no different from what everyone else was dealing with. This isn't the battle of the sexes, it's the battle of the bulge, and we all need help.

Lots of us feel we are alone in our struggles—until we find that so many others contend with exactly the same set of challenges and issues. I began to realize that my own weight story was a very common one and that my own failings—and later on, my victories—were shared by many others. I also began to recognize that my weight gain and loss was in some way a microcosm of what has become an obesity epidemic.

In other words, I am not alone. And neither are you.

Let's beat this thing together.

# Obesity, Then and Now

In 1962, about 13 percent of adult Americans were clinically obese. Today, that number has nearly tripled to 34 percent. Okay, those are adults, and some of them probably picked their own poison. But the tragedy deepens when you think that approximately 17 percent of kids between the ages of 2 and 19 are now classified as clinically obese. How did they reach that state?

In 1990, there were 10 states with obesity prevalence rates below 10 percent, and no state had an obesity rate worse than 15 percent. By 2010, there was not a single state in the country with an obesity level below 20 percent, and 12 states had obesity rates in excess of 30 percent. Today, Colorado is the thinnest state in the Union. A testimony to fresh air, tall peaks, and John Denver, you say? Consider that it would be by far the heaviest state by 1990 standards. This is not a gradual change occurring over centuries. This is a radical 20-year shift—a tectonic plate moving across the dinner table toward you. And me.

## THE HEALTH IMPLICATIONS ARE DISASTROUS

When my company, Weight Watchers, was founded in 1963, people (that is, women) lost weight to look better and to feel in control. Weight Watchers was in the business of personal improvement.

The connection between obesity and health has only gained widespread acknowledgment since the 1990s. Over the past

10 years, and particularly the past 3, the obesity alarm bells have started clanging with real urgency. We now know that obesity causes or exacerbates a host of health issues, including:

Coronary heart disease
Type 2 diabetes
Certain forms of cancer (breast, colon, endometrial)
Hypertension (high blood pressure)
Dyslipidemia (high total cholesterol or triglyceride levels)
Stroke
Liver and gallbladder disease
Sleep apnea
Osteoarthritis
Infertility

Let's take one of the biggest examples, type 2 diabetes. In 1970, about 5 percent of Americans had diabetes. Today, 11 percent have it. By 2050, the Centers for Disease Control and Prevention (CDC) estimates that one-third of us will have it. How do they know? Right now, an estimated 78 million Americans have prediabetes. And there are ominous signs among younger generations. For years, type 2 diabetes was referred to as adult-onset diabetes because only grown-ups were afflicted. With an alarming number of children now suffering from this condition, the health care community was forced to drop the "adult-onset" part.

What is driving this alarming rate of growth in diabetes? Part of it is that we've gotten better at diagnosing the disease. Also, people with the condition are being treated, so they live longer with it and continue showing up on the CDC stat sheets. But the biggest driver of type 2 diabetes is obesity. Someone with a BMI greater than 30 (i.e., clinically obese, right in the crosshairs, as I was a decade ago) has a 500 percent greater chance of ending up with diabetes than someone with a BMI at 25 or less.

For these folks, diabetes isn't the only threat. A clinically obese person—hello, David of 1999!—is 300 percent more likely to die from heart disease than someone living at a healthy weight.

I squeaked out of the death and diabetes demo. Will the rest of us be so lucky?

# THE COST IMPLICATIONS ARE EVEN WORSE

As a nation, we now spend about $2.5 trillion a year on health care costs, which consume about 18 percent of our GDP. It is estimated that by the year 2018, we will be spending $4.4 trillion, or 20 percent of our GDP, on health care. Of the money *now* spent on health care, about 75 percent goes to the treatment of chronic diseases, including heart disease, cancer, pulmonary troubles, diabetes, and other tales of woe. Depending on the condition, 50 to 80 percent of chronic disease is driven by lifestyle, including smoking, obesity, lack of exercise, stress, and otherwise living like I did in my twenties. These factors are driving most of the increases in health care costs.

Rising health care costs increase pressure on programs such as Medicare and Medicaid along with insurance premiums. Over the past 10 years, the average premiums for private health insurance plans have increased at nearly 8 percent per year. The result of rising Medicare and Medicaid costs is increasing federal spending and therefore deficits. The result of rising insurance premiums is increasing pressure on wages and greater out-of-pocket costs for individuals and employees.

So how much of this economic quagmire can be laid on the doorstep of obesity? In CDC-funded research in 2009, obesity costs in the United States accounted for about 9 percent of total health care costs. A few fun statistics to illuminate the impact:

- Obese adults in the United States spent 42 percent more for medical care in 2006 than their healthy weight counterparts.
- Every unit of BMI over 25 increases medical costs and drug costs by approximately $200 and $83, respectively, per person per year.

- Obesity is estimated to cost the country $147 billion per year in 2008 dollars.
- Obesity costs to US employers are estimated to be $13 billion per year.

Enough of this. Economics is the dismal science; the economics of obesity are the dismalest of all. In short, the way we live is threatening to bankrupt our health care system, limit our prosperity, and make us generally miserable at the same time. Have we had enough, finally?

# And Now, for Some Good News

We do not need to look like swimsuit models to significantly improve our health and stop the obesity epidemic. While it is true that health risks are lowest when BMI falls to 25 or below, substantial health benefits come from simply losing 10 percent of our excess baggage. Lose that 10 percent and keep it off, and the following lovely prizes are yours to keep:

- Reducing the likelihood of type 2 diabetes by more than 50 percent
- Reducing lifetime medical expenses by $2,200 to $5,300 (you could spend it on skinny jeans, for instance)
- Reducing systolic blood pressure (the top number) of 6.1 mmHg
- Increasing life expectancy by 2 to 7 months (for me at my heaviest, that would work out to 9 extra days of living per pound lost; I'd do that deal in a minute!)

Let's put 10 percent weight loss in perspective. The average woman who joins Weight Watchers in the United States is about 5 foot 4 and weighs roughly 199 pounds. This is a BMI of 34—clinically obese. Losing 10 percent of her weight would be 20 pounds, bringing her down to 179. She'd still be clinically obese, but she would have reduced her risk of getting diabetes by 59 percent! She'd feel better every day of her life, have more energy, and richly earn the shopping spree to buy clothes to fit her new body.

So our challenge as a society, at Weight Watchers, and individually is not to create bikini models, but rather to help one another achieve medically meaningful weight loss. No, we can't all be Marissa Miller, jetting off to the islands for a *Sports Illustrated* cover shoot. If we can shift our focus and simply concentrate on achieving a more realistic reduction in a sustainable way, we can win this fight collectively and as individuals.

# But We're Not Out of the Woods Yet

None of this is easy to do. There are lots of ways to lose weight, and we've all tried one or more of them. How many of us have lost weight, regained it, lost it, and regained it again?

We blame ourselves for our food failures, for our lack of willpower. But it's not your fault. Heck, I've forgiven myself for my many transgressions. That's because I've learned that, to address obesity, we need to understand what has caused it. In fact, you and I haven't changed that radically, but our environment and life circumstances have.

Really, the causes of obesity are fairly well understood. We citizens of the modern world do not move around nearly as much as our forebears did. Most of us have desk jobs, and we spend a lot more time sitting in front of the TV and in cars instead of playing outside, doing manual labor, or using our feet for transportation. We are also surrounded by a lot more food, most of it processed with lots of added sugars and fats. We are much more likely to eat out than to cook a meal at home. On top of our slowdown, our portion sizes have accelerated past the edges of our plates and overflowed our plastic cups.

This is what experts refer to as our obesogenic society.

We now live in an environment that encourages us to eat too much of the wrong foods while we simultaneously burn fewer calories. The net effect of this is about an extra 200 calories per day added to our bottom lines, and that's all you need to create an obesity epidemic.

There are other problems as well. Some people are more genetically predisposed to obesity than others. And there is research to indicate that our metabolisms slow as we lose weight, which can make keeping weight off that much more difficult.

All of these challenges are very real, and some of them are very difficult, but what's our alternative? Do we give up on ourselves as adults? Resign ourselves to a world in which our children follow in our heavy footsteps? Of course not. But we can use these challenges as a catalyst to make sure that we are using the full set of tools to turn back the fat tide that's threatening to engulf us.

# There Has to Be a Better Way ...

Before we get to that, I owe you an answer to a question you may be pondering: Why another book on weight loss? On a recent trip to Barnes & Noble, I counted about five shelves full of them.

I don't think any of them will be quite like this one. So many books and articles on weight focus on what foods to eat, while little effort is expended on explaining how to create a sustainable healthy lifestyle. In some respects, what to eat is the least complicated part of a sustainable weight loss process, which can be summed up in these five simple guidelines:

- Eat vegetables, fruits, lean proteins, whole grains, and low-fat dairy.
- Avoid junk food.
- Watch portion size.

- Exercise daily.
- Repeat.

Okay, there's a little more to it than that. But if you look at most scientifically based diets, from Ornish to South Beach, they pretty much stick to these five basic rules.

The challenging part is hitting all five—*forever*. This requires forming new healthy habits and routines while eliminating bad ones. It requires a combination of both better food choices and regular exercise. It requires repetition and practice. It requires a new mind-set. It requires behavior change.

Behavior change is not for the faint of heart. While quitting smoking is famously difficult, it's also binary: You do it or you don't. That's not the case with good nutrition. All of us eat for reasons that have nothing to do with being hungry. We eat because we are sad, happy, bored, busy, anxious, or relaxed. We use food as a reward or as medication. And exercise is subject to all sorts of conditions, from the weather to your aching knee joint. It makes touching match to cancer-causing tobacco product seem ridiculously simple, by comparison.

So again, why this book? Here's my answer: In the process of writing my regular blog posts, pulling in science and health observations, and being surrounded by the topic of weight 24/7 (from my job and from my own tendency to add pounds), I have formed my own set of opinions about proactive ways to address a weight issue. I'm not a scientist in a lab or a celeb on TV. But I have wrestled with weight as a person and as a professional, so I just might have a unique perspective on my own weight and yours.

I want to share my own experience of gaining weight, losing weight, and, most important, holding firm against a return to larger pants. What we now know about weight maintenance is critical to helping us lose weight in the first place. My life has been changed immeasurably for the better, so I'm driven to share that experience. I know many others who have shared the same kinds of epiphanies I've had, and there's strength and knowledge in our numbers.

But you can learn a lot from my failures, too. I certainly have. My experiences may not be the same as yours, and my exact approach may also differ. In fact, I'm sure it will. When we train our Weight Watchers staff, we tell each of them the same thing: "We are the experts in weight management, but each member is the expert on himself or herself." You know what your pitfalls are and where you're at your best. I'm hoping that, by talking through my own weight loss trials, and ultimate (knock on wood) triumph, I can help you craft your own great story. But by working at Weight Watchers and spending countless hours listening to people share their life and loss histories, I now know that we are much more alike than we are different.

Everywhere I go, people ask me what they should do to lose weight. I'm not shy about advising them, just as other, smarter people have advised me. This book gives me a chance to elaborate on the key points I've used myself and seen work for other people like me. Know this: It's about not living in deprivation. It's about establishing habits and mastering your environment. (No more fun-size Snickers stashed in the freezer, you hear?)

There is a lot to discuss in these pages, but here's what I'm going to focus on:

# THE 5 KEY THEMES OF THIS BOOK

**1.** Establishing healthy habits and routines while getting rid of (or at least minimizing) the bad habits

**2.** Learning how to master our obesogenic environment and taking control

**3.** Eating smarter to avoid feelings of deprivation

**4.** Shifting exercise into automatic (you are a machine; we just need to find your "on" switch)

**5.** Succeeding in maintenance: making a healthy life sustainable

Scientific research and expert sources (including people who have inspired me by losing weight and keeping it off) will help you understand and implement these key themes. After each chapter, you'll meet those inspirations in a series of Weight Watchers Profiles and learn from them as I have. I draw a lot from my experience working at Weight Watchers, but this book is not intended only or even primarily for people following our PointsPlus® program. Regardless of how you approach weight management, these themes are applicable. If I get bogged down in Weight Watchers–speak, bear with me; I promise to provide a decoder ring for the key phrases.

Likewise, I'll present a fair amount of research evidence, if only to show my scientist dad that I wasn't napping through my expensive coursework at Duke. But you should also know this: The science of weight loss is relatively young. More discoveries are being made every year, expanding our understanding of how the body and mind work together to make us who we are. They can work for better or worse—and *nobody* has the final word on what those processes are or how we can manipulate them. We're refining what we know; it's an evolution of knowledge, not a revolution.

It frustrates me as a person with weight challenges that there just aren't answers to every question. But by seeking your own personal answers—maybe with the help of a formerly chubby CEO who's hanging on to his weight loss gains by his fingernails—you're already making progress.

I will bring these themes to life by relating them to my own experiences and those of people who have succeeded even more than I have. Bear with me if some of my examples (including an entire chapter) are somewhat type A and overly full of testosterone. Get past the bravado, and you will find me to be firmly in touch with my feminine side. Also, I hope you'll bear with my oddities and my failings. If you can laugh with and at me along the way, all the better! I'm happy to be the comic relief in the drama of your self-reinvention. The plot will have twists and turns, of course, but the ending will be magnificent. Less hips, more happy!

# The Unofficial Weight Watchers Decoder Ring

As noted several times, this book was never intended to be about following the Weight Watchers program. I obviously talk about it a lot because (1) I work there, (2) I think it's pretty great (I'm understandably biased), and (3) it's how I lost my weight and how I'm keeping it off. You definitely do not need to follow Weight Watchers to practice most of what is covered in the pages that follow. However, there will be times you will have to deal with my jargon and insider terms. So to help take some of the mystery out, here are some of the basics of Weight Watchers as well as some terms you might stumble across.

## WEIGHT WATCHERS BASICS

The current Weight Watchers program is called PointsPlus (it's called ProPoints outside of North America). The most basic elements of the program are the following:

- Every food is assigned a PointsPlus value that is calculated from the grams of protein, fat, carbohydrates, and fiber in a defined portion of the food.

- Fruits and nonstarchy vegetables are assigned a PointsPlus value of zero, although we never encourage eating 12 bananas at a time or in a day, for a whole bunch of reasons.

- Some foods are called Weight Watchers Power Foods because they are a great PointsPlus bargain, are naturally filling, and have good nutritional characteristics.

- You can earn additional PointsPlus values from exercise. The more the exercise makes you work, the more Activity PointsPlus values you can earn and then swap (or not) for food.

- Each person is assigned a PointsPlus Target to live within each day. To provide additional flexibility, we also provide something called a Weekly Allowance, which allows you to splurge on occasion. Some, none, or all of the allowance can be used each week.

People who attend Weight Watchers do it primarily through one of two routes.

• **Meetings:** Where you actually go to a meeting place at a retail location, your office, or a community location such as a community center. At these meetings, there is a leader who is a successful member and now works for Weight Watchers. This person facilitates a discussion around a selected topic as well as a discussion on how everyone is doing. At these meetings, people get weigh-ins, which are performed confidentially by a receptionist, who is also a successful Weight Watchers member.

• **Weight Watchers Online:** Where you use an array of Web-based tools and resources and/or mobile applications to learn the PointsPlus program and track your food consumption and weight loss progress.

Most people who go to meetings these days purchase a Monthly Pass, which gives them unlimited access to meetings, and the online tools, as well as any mobile applications.
    Other terms you might stumble across:

• **Goal weight:** Fairly self-explanatory, except that Weight Watchers focuses heavily in the first few months on achieving medically significant weight loss, which occurs when you lose 5 to 10 percent of your weight.

• **Lifetime Membership:** Members who reach a BMI of 25 (or higher with a doctor's note) and maintain it for 6 weeks are eligible for Lifetime Membership. This special status allows them to continue going to meetings for free as long as they stay within 2 pounds of their goal weight and weigh in once a month.

There is much more to the program than this, but this gives you a very general lay of the land.

# PART I
# From Thin to Heavy and Back Again:
## A Weight Loss Odyssey

# {CHAPTER 1}
# Paging Dr. Freud—
## Early Influences and Food Attitudes

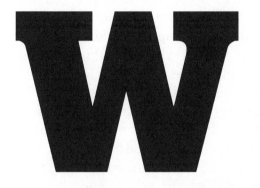 HEN I LOOK at
the latest version of
Windows, I can't help
but see the influences,
features, and DNA
traces of all the ver-
sions that preceded it.
If I look hard enough,
I can even detect
glimmers of MS-DOS
kicking around, and nobody wants to see that. I think of my
own brain as a compendium of code that's been written,
overwritten, rewritten, appended, corrupted, and patched
with a frightening number of version upgrades and perfor-
mance patches.

Don't worry, I'm not pulling out random comparisons
between my brain and the most profitable (annoying?) piece
of software in world history. One of the important lessons
I have learned at Weight Watchers International—and during
my own 25-year weight loss journey—is that biography really
is the key to behavior. Many of my first personal operating
systems are still up and running; I hear the grinding of the
hard drive when I look at why I eat, how I eat, how I think
about my body, how I see myself, and how I handle temptation. David Kirchhoff 1.0 (beta) is always going to be lurking
in my circuitry no matter how many times I try to purge,
upgrade, or defrag. Therefore, I have some choices.

- I can completely ignore the early programming that led to my current crashes.

- I can troubleshoot that antiquated code to help get past my many glitches.

- I can make smart upgrades when better programming becomes available.

For me, this is the paradox of childhood. (And I'll drop the computer metaphor now, in memory of Steve Jobs.) Our early years are a massive influence on who we are, and yet we're not bound by these influences. I optimistically believe that they can be harnessed to help us achieve what we need to. For instance, if I understand my deep-seated urge to blow through a half gallon of ice cream at a single sitting, I can learn from it. If I know that these forces are kicking around whether I want them to or not, then I can cut myself a break when I crawl under the barbed wire to escape my healthy living ranch. I also know that willpower alone isn't enough to triumph over these urges. Half gallons are the enemy; I keep them out of spoon range.

All of this is another way of saying: I cannot change my future if I do not understand my past.

# From Skinny Jeans to Fat Genes

I became the CEO of Weight Watchers International in January 2007 after assuming a bunch of different roles at the company over the previous 7 years. Never in a thousand years could I have imagined myself in this line of work, and I certainly did not start my life as a Weight Watchers guy.

I was born on August 20, 1966, to William H. Kirchhoff and Ann R. Kirchhoff, at George Washington University Hospital in Washington, DC. I was the third of four kids in my family with an older sister, Meg (by 7 years), an older brother, Dan (by 5 years), and a younger sister, Jenny (by 4 years).

My father worked as a basic research scientist, specializing in chemical physics with a focus on thermodynamics. He spent his career principally at the National Bureau of Standards and then the Department of Energy, where he oversaw the awarding of grants to scientists in academic research centers. (Hmmmm. National standards, energy regulation—sounds like what I do for a living now!)

My mother started her grown-up life at Carleton College before transferring to the University of Illinois to be with my dad (they started dating in high school in Downers Grove, Illinois). My mom taught school for a few years while my dad earned his doctorate in chemistry at Harvard. When he landed his first job, she stayed home and took care of her offspring.

My parents were both the first in their respective families to get college degrees. Trying my best to maintain the family win streak, I worked pretty hard in high school to get into a good college, Duke, where I focused on a self-taught tutorial on beer drinking. I applied myself to nondrinking activities during grad school at the University of Chicago, and I surprised myself by getting good grades. Maybe it just took that long for my parents' good example to penetrate through layers of skull.

Okay, so now you know what was going on upstairs. How about around my midsection?

Here is the first important fact about my childhood: I was insanely skinny. I'm half surprised that my inwardly facing belly button didn't poke out of my back.

Let's start with a few physical observations about myself.

- I grew tall fast, and not in a particularly graceful, NBA-player-waiting-to-happen kind of way. I was all arms and legs, equipped with little coordination for most of my preadult life.

- I topped out at 6 foot 3 during high school, but I only managed to pack 170 pounds onto my frame, even though

I was built from farming stock. The only cultivation job I qualified for was "scarecrow." Throw on a respectable case of acne, and you've got the visual of Teen-David.

This raises a few questions: If I later had, and on some level still have, a weight problem, why was I so skinny growing up? Why didn't I just stay skinny? Shouldn't I be a naturally skinny person? What other impacts did my childhood have on my weight, including those that ultimately led to weight gain?

The genetics of weight is fascinating and is an area of study that's growing by leaps and bounds. It's been known for a long time that heavy parents are more likely to have heavy kids than thin ones. One long-term study, tracing people from the 1950s to the 1980s, showed that the odds of becoming an obese adult

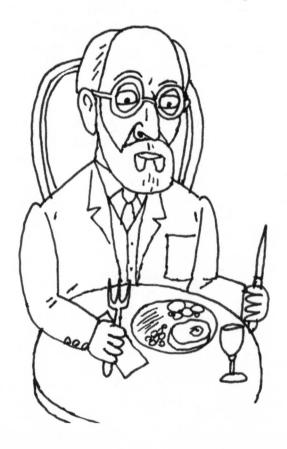

if you grew up during these decades were high to start with, but they were even higher if your parents were obese.

Understanding the role that family life plays in weight is complex. We are a product of both our genes and the home environment in which we were raised. Moreover, recent research is revealing that these two factors—genes and environment—can influence the odds of being an obese adult from the moment of conception, to birth, through childhood, and even into adulthood. That's one reason why there are such wildly divergent estimates— anywhere from 5 to 90 percent— in assessing the impact of genes on weight. Among identical twins, 50 to 70 percent of their adult weight can be traced to heredity. When looking at the entire population, genetics accounts for 40 to 50 percent of what we weigh. Just how much heredity accounts for your weight—and you're the most important person we address in this book—is a product of the genetic tossed salad you were born with.

To further complicate the gene story, newer research is finding that the influence of genetics goes beyond vulnerability for weight gain, obesity, and body fat. Our weight-related behaviors (things like food cravings, taste preferences, and propensity to be physically active) also carry some interesting genetic links and influences. Stay tuned, folks, as this is a new scientific frontier.

Which makes its usefulness somewhat of a question. One day, we'll be able to use genetic research to help fine-tune a weight management program, but we are not quite there yet. The other way to look at it is this: If you know you are genetically predisposed, then there is all the more reason to be careful and protect yourself in this dangerous food world we currently inhabit. You can't choose your parents, but you can choose how you live, and virtually every study attests to a strong link between weight and lifestyle. Seize the opportunity there, because it's your best chance to wrest control of the scale from your parents, your DNA, and other ghosts in the machine.

# More to Eat–And Gain

Why is it that in the 1970s, about 15 percent of adult Americans were obese while today more than 30 percent are? A report published in *The Lancet* comparing trends in activity expenditure and food consumption over the past 100 years found that obesity rates stayed in check from 1910 to 1970, despite the fact that our increasingly "mechanized" and "motorized" society was becoming more sedentary (the amount of available food actually *decreased* somewhat). Then, starting in the 1970s, as new grocery items containing sugars and fats proliferated, the amount of food in the US supply chain jumped by 600 calories per day, boosting total energy consumption (measured in "kilojoules")—and obesity.

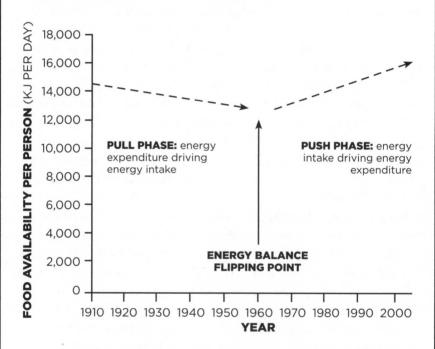

That's not to say we've been munching all 600 calories per day; the real number for the average American is closer to 200 calories, as some of that food goes to waste. But that little bit extra may have been enough to tip the scales!

# MY LEAN ENVIRONMENT: THE EARLY YEARS

If obesity was purely a function of genetics, there would be no clear explanation for the fact that obesity rates have been sky-rocketing over the past 30 years. As noted, much of what has been driving obesity has been the rapid change in the food and activity environment around us, and this environmental influence is pretty self-evident: If there were no calorie-dense foods around us, then we would not eat them. Therefore, part of the challenge before us is how to recreate our personal food and exercise environments (i.e., in our homes and offices) in order to craft a workable healthy lifestyle. Lifestyle simply refers to the choices we make in our daily lives, compensating for the underlying triggers that drive our behaviors—eating because we're sad, happy, bored, anxious, or any number of other emotional reasons.

I've spent a lot of time thinking about how I grew so heavy, but it's also instructive to think about what kept me so skinny during those early years. Certainly some of it was my faster metabolism. But I think my weight back then had much more to do with the way I was fed and the food available in my house.

In short: It all comes back to my mom.

It goes without saying that my food environment has changed pretty radically from when I was a kid. Back then, it looked more like the Gobi Desert than the Garden of Eating. But my feelings of deprivation led me to bust out in a fierce way once my food environment became unconstrained. I didn't binge eat much because there was nothing to binge on. Here's my typical meal plan while I was growing up.

- **Breakfast:** cereal and skim milk (reconstituted powdered skim milk at that)

- **Lunch:** cheese and mustard sandwich, banana, and 6 ounces of chocolate milk; no extra treat

- **Dinner:** normal portions of whatever my mom cooked that night, served on a plate that would seem laughably small by today's standards

- **Dessert:** a treat, once a week; usually low-fat ice cream (then known as ice milk) served with a 12-ounce soda

What about restaurants? We went to McDonald's four to six times per year, so as you might guess, every single visit was a spectacular, glorious event. We went to a nice restaurant on my birthday, and every once in a while my parents would order Chinese food or pizza. We loved restaurants, but a hard-working government scientist had neither the time nor the money to treat his family of six very often.

And what about the great big drawer in the kitchen filled with chips, crackers, and cookies? Not in my house. Sneaking treats in my house was about as fun as being the mouse in the pantry at Bob Cratchit's house. The cupboard was bare.

I couldn't make spectacularly bad food decisions because there was nothing around to tempt me. So what did I do about food as a young lad? Simple. I ate at mealtimes, consuming normal and healthy portions of food. I didn't snack much or eat fast food. So I stayed really skinny until I left my perfectly controlled anti-obesogenic environment and landed in the free-for-all known as college.

I'm mentioning all of this not just to give my mom a hard time for starving me. It's also because she came up with the solution to the obesogenic nightmare before it had even been given a name. Her implicit strategy: Don't go near that stuff.

The way I see it, I have two choices: I can focus my energy on developing mental muscle power to withstand the temptations of a food-dense environment all around me; or I can manage my environment, so I won't be tested constantly.

My mom had the answer, and it's simple: If there is little tempting, there is little temptation.

Maybe she did it on purpose—looking past my skinny frame to the raging beast within. And I will be the first to admit that

I suffer from food lust, which sometimes feels uncontrollable. When the beast escapes, he engages in mindless eating, binge consumption, and lurid food fantasies.

So you know, I think the world of my mom. She didn't have much to work with when it came to me, and I turned out pretty okay. But it is impossible to parent without inflicting at least two or three unforeseen consequences on your offspring. I'm certainly guilty with my kids, just as she was probably guilty with me. If you could call it that. Her "sins" may actually have saved me.

My mom was a born saver. Her parents struggled through the Great Depression, and she and my dad never had much money when they were starting out in the world as adults. Somehow her bone-deep frugality found its most extreme expression in the food in our house.

A few notable examples come to mind.

- **The wrong bags:** Other kids got those cool precut lunch bags made explicitly for carrying their lunch to school. I got whatever large brown shopping bag happened to be around. I looked like a street urchin in search of canned goods.

- **Stale bread:** We never got fresh bread from the store. Instead, we stocked up on day-old bread on sale and stored it in our industrial-size freezer. I didn't complain as bitterly as my siblings, so I got the heels, not the normal slices from the middle. That's right. My sandwiches were made out of day-old frozen-then-thawed heel slices. It wasn't even Wonder Bread! Generic all the way.

- **Cheez? Please!** Did I get those awesome-tasting processed cheese slices that the cool kids got? Nope. Bologna? Never! I got store-brand Cheddar splooshed with mustard. Some days, I did get PB&J, but no sign of Mr. Peanut or Skippy. It was generic or nothing.

- **Disappointing "treat":** Usually a brown banana. I was the kid who had nothing good to trade at lunch in the cafeteria. I was at the end of the food chain, with no way up.

- **Unlucky charms:** Okay, lunch was sad, but what about breakfast? Anything tasty and sweet on the menu? No. In those days, Safeway sold a private label that was literally a white box with black letters bearing catchy derivative names like "Oats of Cheery." We were early participants in the cult of private labels. No Lucky Charms for this boy.

- **Astronaut milk:** To this day, I find this hard to believe. We bought the huge box of powdered skim milk. My mom said it was just like what the astronauts had! Sure, ones who were visiting a dry, tasteless, dusty planet. I don't think I tasted fresh whole milk until I was 16 years old.

- **Not-so-awful dinner:** My mom was a good cook, so this was the culinary highlight. The portions were small, but we divided up what we had, and nobody complained.

- **The rare dessert:** One night each week, I got the "Treat of the Week." It was usually a Black Cow, which was private label ice milk plopped into store label root beer.

There you have it: the feast at Casa de Kirchhoff. It kept me alive until I escaped the house, but the moments of pleasure were few and far between. I still ask myself: Was that a bad thing or a good thing?

How did it affect my attitudes toward food? I was envious of kids who had the branded processed foods and had frequent access to fast food. Though they lived in the epicenter of our obesogenic world, all I could think of back then was that they had the good life. I felt like a poor kid wearing my Sears Toughskins jeans, carrying my big brown shopping bag with a crusty cheese sandwich and a brown banana.

To this day, my palms sweat when I see brand-name food. A lot of people are label conscious with clothes; I feel that way about Doritos. I still cannot stand the idea of buying generic food. Why? The most expensive food must certainly be of higher quality. Right? Logically, I know that's not true, but my belly rumbles in disagreement.

Listen, I know now that I grew up in relatively privileged circumstances. My parents loved me, and I didn't want for anything that was truly essential. But I felt the need to rebel against the lean times at my house. For me, there is still something comforting about being able to buy and eat any food I want, whenever I want it. You can see how my need to prove that to myself, over and over, can lead to far too many meals out, too many burgers consumed, too much "all you can eat" reassurance.

In retrospect, I know my mother created a healthy environment for her kids. Maybe my mom was just ahead of her time. But I do think that I formed a link between my Oliver Twist existence—craving more, afraid to ask for it—and the social status and wealth indicators that I so badly wanted. I desperately wanted to fit in with the mainstream of my school, even if that mainstream was flowing with deep fat from the fryers.

So that's the story of how one man developed an unhealthy relationship with food. It had nothing to do with food itself, but rather my own perception of social worth and acceptance. Strange, isn't it?

# LIKE FATHER, LIKE SON

I'm blaming much of my desire for brand-name calorie-dense foods on my poor mother, but what about my dad? He's much less agile than my mother and is therefore less able to dodge my attacks. There must be something in my unhealthy habit inventory that I can lay on his doorstep.

Ah, there it is. Ice cream. Can the sins of the father be passed along to the son? I say: most definitely, especially when it comes studded with frozen M&Ms.

My mom and dad came through one weekend to watch my older daughter perform in her middle school play (she was excellent, BTW). We were having a normal Saturday morning coffee chat when we started talking about the blog post where I heaped blame on my mom. We talked about how weird food habits seemed to be formed at a young age. They both talked about the fact that I was a chronic food sneaker even as a little kid. Their favorite story: Once upon a time there was a remarkable seven-year-old boy named David (okay, the "remarkable" was my contribution), and Mom and Dad were preparing to go out for the evening. They had not quite closed the door to leave the house when they heard their son call out: "Hey guys, Mom and Dad are gone. Let's sneak!"

Fine. Guilty as charged. I was a seven-year-old food larcenist. Apparently, I was not a particularly stealthy one. My folks have gotten more mileage out of that than the VW bug they drove for much of my childhood.

But I still wonder: Why was I a food sneak? Why do I still feel the temptation to snitch a cookie here, snarf a bagful of horrors there?

Oh, how convenient: Here's my dad, and he has a confession to make.

My dad admitted that he still raids the ice cream coffers when nobody is around. If ice cream is in the house, it is unsafe. (If we're both in the house with a half gallon, it's double jeopardy.)

Admit it: Lots of us sneak.

Within families, some of us are a pair of sneakers. My dad and I match, right down to the silent tread on the kitchen floor as we approach the freezer, spoon in hand.

It's hard for me to be mad at the guy, though. When I watch him, I see someone who truly loves food. That is, I see myself. We've both got some work to do. And if my description of my ice cream sneak attack sent you to the freezer—I saw you!— then you've got work to do, too.

We'll pitch in together, just a few chapters ahead. But first . . .

# SOME OTHER RELATIVES (AND FOOD TENDENCIES) THAT I FRANKLY JUST DON'T UNDERSTAND

Another adult who had a pretty significant impact on my life was my grandmother on my mother's side, Mary. Grandma Mary passed away about 8 years ago after an incredibly full 89 years. As noted earlier, Mary was a product of the Great Depression. She remembered that, during those rough times, she and her family gave out apples to people who simply had nothing to eat. There were no safety nets back then, and 25 percent unemployment took a terrible toll on too many people to count. People who grew up then look at money in a very different way.

Mary was one of those people.

Whereas I suffer from food lust, a gift from my otherwise excellent father, Mary was a model of propriety. When we would visit her in Cape Cod, we could count on excellent food that was delivered in precisely the correct proportions. If there was dessert, it was a piece of spice cake that would cube out at 1.5 square inches max. More often, she spooned out homemade fruit salad. Rations were thin—in both senses of the word—during those summer visits to the Cape. Grandma Mary was one of those people who ate to live rather than lived to eat.

She also made a ritual of exercise, walking pretty much every day for at least a mile, until she got cancer at the age of 87. She got much more pleasure out of moving around than she ever seemed to get from sitting down to a meal.

When I was a younger man, she made me feel somewhat inadequate. I envied her discipline and certitude, plus her abundant character when it came to taking care of herself. Deep down, I think I might have even resented her a bit while also wanting her approval.

With the passing of time, I can now see her as much more of a role model. She was a naturally disciplined person who developed a set of life rituals—the walk in the morning, cutting up fruit for the salad—that took the decision making out of living healthfully. The more she repeated them, the better she looked and felt.

In my saner health moments, I have strived to live a lot more like my grandmother. If she were still around today, she would in fact approve—and then ask me if I want to go for a walk.

# Find Your Inner
# Weight Loss Boss

## Understand how early conditions can come back to haunt you later

## Note to self: It's the environment, stupid!

By merely examining the changing nature of our environment, we can take steps to significantly improve the likelihood that we can stick with a healthier lifestyle. If there is not a ton of junk in the house, then there is no junk to eat. I'm not ready to return to 1972 (the TV was too small), but the fact is that the more my house looks like my mother's house, the better off my family and I are.

## Know your early influences and weak spots.

I do enjoy teasing my mom and dad, but that doesn't mean they're guilty of anything I ascribe to them. It is important, however, for me to recognize that my relationship with food goes back to some pretty deep-rooted influences. I really doubt whether some of these impulses will ever go away. Even more, I am probably doing myself a disservice by pretending this early wiring does not exist anymore. It does exist. Knowing this allows me to:

- Understand that I tend to lose it around food
- Recognize my impulses and deal with them
- Put myself in situations where I can avoid fights with my vestigial DOS drive (I will lose many of these battles, so it's better to avoid fighting them in the first place).

## Weight Watchers Profile

### "When I sing 'Feeling Good,' that's for real!"

The "Dream Girl" reaches her dream weight

**Jennifer Hudson,** *Chicago, IL*

**LOST:** Baby fat, mom fat
**FOUND:** New confidence on the red carpet

#### MY STRUGGLE

I come from the South Side of Chicago, where a lot of girls have curves. Food was a central focus for all types of gatherings, from family reunions to Sunday night dinners. As I got older, all of those big meals, plus junk food, began to catch up with me. By the time I was in my teens, I was aware that I had become a plus-size girl.

#### MY WAKE-UP CALL

In the fall of 2008, I had started a new weight loss regimen, and I noticed I was feeling unusually tired. I decided to take a home pregnancy test just to rule it out. I looked down. Positive. Pregnant. I suddenly went from thinking for myself to thinking like a mama in 30 seconds flat. I was shocked that even after giving birth, I still weighed around 237

pounds. This was the biggest number I had seen on the scale in many years.

I agreed to give Weight Watchers a try. After my first week, I lost 5 pounds. With that result, I actually wanted to stick to their program.

#### MY FOOD

Although I was already a pretty healthy eater, I was making tiny mistakes that were throwing me off and keeping my weight loss stagnant. I realized that portion control and lack of awareness were my two biggest challenges.

While I don't have a set weekly menu, I do have some favorites that have helped me get to my goal. A typical breakfast for me became one of three meals: grilled chicken breast fajitas with brown rice, an egg-white omelet with smoked salmon, or a chicken and vegetable omelet. I go for the real thing. If I want orange sherbet, I'll reach for an orange instead of the ice cream. It's the flavor I'm going for, so why not eat something that has fiber and nutrients over something that is full of chemicals and artificial flavors?

**MY FITNESS**

My workouts are never the same. Some days I run outside or sprint up hills in our local park, while others I'd rather use the treadmill at the gym. On the road, I exercise to DVDs. I like to run up and down stairs, too. I figure that as long as I am moving, I am burning calories.

**MY PAYOFF**

Nothing prepared me for the attention I now get as a result of losing weight. Walking the red carpet has taken on a whole new dimension. I get to stand next to the skinny supermodel talking about what I am wearing, about my eyelashes, earrings, and even the color of my toenail polish! Years ago, the only thing anyone wanted to talk about was if I felt insecure as a big girl in Hollywood.

I've always been comfortable with my size, but I haven't always felt healthy like I do now. After I discovered the positivity in my new and healthier body, I began to notice that I wanted to surround myself with other positive people, too. An organic shift began to take place in my entire life. As my weight loss progressed, I shared my newfound love for healthy eating with my sister and my family. Altogether, 75 of my family members have gone on the program and they have collectively lost more than 2,000 pounds. Allowing myself to be overweight and unhealthy is a habit I've gladly left in my past—I've got more energy, stamina, and drive than I've ever had. When I am singing "Feeling Good" in my Weight Watchers commercials, that's for real. They couldn't have picked a better song to describe where I am on the journey. And if I can do it, anyone can.

Excerpted from *I Got This: How I Changed My Ways and Lost What Weighed Me Down,* by Jennifer Hudson (Dutton).

# {CHAPTER 2}

# Letting Loose

## in an Obesogenic Environment

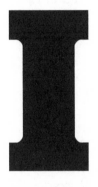**T'S PRETTY TYPICAL FOR GUYS TO GAIN WEIGHT** in their twenties and thirties—a slowing metabolism, a ravenous appetite, and extra chair time will do that to a guy (or girl). The cliché goes like this: Guy plays sports in high school; guy goes to college and collects a used couch, a fresh case of beer, and the phone number for a pizza delivery place; guy has no one around forcing him to curb his appetites, so his belt line begins expanding like it was his manifest destiny.

The question I didn't think to ask before leaving for college was: How would I handle the transition to free-range living? Ironically, my mother was more concerned about another aspect of that transition, imploring me to stay away from hard liquor and to please not create any children out of wedlock. Considering that my parents kept a hammerlock on me until the day I graduated from high school, I found it rather an Evel Knievel–ish leap from "be home by 11 p.m." to "stay away from whiskey and sexual reproduction." It never occurred to my folks to worry about whether I would belly up to the trough and eat myself into a stupor. Surprise! That's exactly what I did.

The college "freshman 15" was way beneath my eating skills. I managed to gain 45 pounds by the end of my freshman year. Impressive! How did I manage to add 25 percent more body weight?

# Welcome to the Cafeteria!

As much as I'd like to blame my freshman 45 on a metabolic change, I doubt that anyone's body chemistry could down-shift quite that quickly. (Not that it stopped me from loudly proclaiming it, however.) Rather, I have sufficient evidence to prove that I was done in by a scintillating range of din-ing options. Duke was the horn of plenty, and my childhood prayers were answered: I was suddenly surrounded by all the food I could possibly want.

As a youngster, I loved cafeterias with every tastebud on my hungry tongue. Some people might be grossed out by the thought of food left too long under heating lamps and served up in giant ladles by women (and men!) with hair-nets. Not me. I can still remember the first time I went to a smorgasbord-themed restaurant. I was about 14, and for a kid who yearned for bad food, it was no-no Nirvana. You could eat as much rubbish as you could cram into your trash-compactor stomach. The seemingly infinite selection of desserts—cherry pie slathered with an everlasting whipped cream–like product, tapioca by the bucket—was beyond my comprehension. (As a side note, how is it that the country that exported the smorgasbord—Sweden—has a mere 9.7 percent obesity rate? Oh, I get it: They sent it over here, then closed the door.)

My freshman year, I majored in smorgasbord. I clearly remember eating gigantic salads heaped with egg fragments (the awesome reconstituted kind), baconlike substances, and at least a cup of blue cheese dressing on top. And then I'd have a burger and fries. And then I had dessert from the soft-serve volcano or the endless pie line. Doing the calculations, I must have been inhaling upward of 4,000 calories a meal, compared with the 2,200 I should have been swallowing daily. I'm lucky I didn't double in size.

How did these all-you-can-eat (AYCE—I needed an acronym, to help speed the feed) orgies induce me and so many others to eat ourselves into near food comas? For me, there seems to be a link between my optic nerve and some kind of trapdoor into my stomach: Pick up a tray and look out below! (And yes, I'm one of those horrible people who will eat food directly from the serving station because my hunger is so profound I'm not certain I'll even make it back to my table.) In contrast, reading a menu has a totally different effect on me. I cannot actually see the food, so I tend to make much saner choices.

Newer research is helping us to understand how and why this happens. Turns out that sensory exposure to palatable foods (or even thinking about them) creates brain signals that say "I want that food now!" Those same signals help muster your motivation to go ahead and kill, and grill, the whole mastodon. The signals appear to be stronger in those who are vulnerable to excess weight—young David says, "That's me! That's me!"—so it's harder to fight them off. But wait, it gets worse: Each new goodie sends out its own set of signals, so the ice cream and the whipped cream and the cherry on top become a choir, singing their siren song to your brain's pleasure pathways. They beckon, you move.

Given the harmonies ringing in my ears, I just kept on opening my mouth, no matter how many times I was disappointed—or even disgusted—by the volumes of food I grabbed at the AYCE feast. My suspicion: The cherry pie is built to look good and last forever, kind of like one of those Egyptian princesses they dig up every now and then. But you wouldn't want to eat one!

I am in fact happy to report that I've finally outgrown my mania over AYCEs. After decades of disappointment, I have trained my brain to recognize that huge displays of shiny food don't deliver the joy I think they will. Now, my tray no longer (okay, rarely) runneth over.

# ANATOMY OF A BEER BELLY

Back when I was in college, the drinking age was 18 or 19, so my right to behave like a drooling buffoon was fully supported by the state legislature in North Carolina. (This comment is inserted in case my kids need to be reminded that the drinking age is now 21 and that I'm watching them every minute. Love you, kids!) Every Thursday night, we tapped kegs at the fraternity; why wait all the way to Friday? In fact, keg-tapping was pretty much an every-night activity, though on the Seventh Night (Sunday) we rested—or were too headachy to even consider anything beer related.

The college itself, an otherwise prestigious academic institution, would regularly allow events where a tractor-trailer would pull up on campus, tap 40 kegs of beer, and supply a band to go with it. Combine the cheap beer landscape with the eat-your-heart-out cafeterias, BBQ joints, and pizza parlors, and every other high-calorie food imaginable, and it is no wonder I burst out of my frame.

I had forgotten to what extent my college beer consumption had impacted my eating habits until about a year ago, when I had the opportunity to do a market visit for Weight Watchers in the Research Triangle area of North Carolina. I arrived the night of the NCAA basketball tournament final. For the uninitiated, that day is to beer what St. Paddy's Day is to green—an excuse to indulge. My Blue Devils had already been eliminated, and our rivals at UNC were out as well. Time to drown sorrows in Amber Fizzy Liquid!

I called on an old friend and fraternity brother who now lives in the Chapel Hill area to watch Butler play UConn in the final. We saddled up in a traditional Chapel Hill college bar, Top of the Hill. I began gingerly picking at a nice piece of salmon served over cheese grits. Just like old times, only with far better food. But, uh-oh, more disposable income. Things started to turn ugly as the well-meaning bartender began treating my beer glass as if it were bottomless. He was probably thinking, "I'll give these old guys one more taste of college life." That was exactly the problem.

The next morning, I had a headache that felt like it had been delivered by a rusty ice pick. I knew the cure for this, because I'd resorted to it too many times while in college: two parts pulled pork BBQ (Eastern style), one part Brunswick stew, with therapeutic doses of baked beans and hush puppies. Just like old times.

So does beer make you fat? In a word, yes (or at least likely). Beer obviously has calories, but it also has the ability to radically lower eating inhibitions while under the influence. Hangovers also require excess food consumption. All of this reminds me of the wise words of the leader of my own Weight Watchers meetings. She tells us: Friends don't let friends eat drunk. Words to live by for any young collegiate buffoon.

As many a dieter can testify, alcohol and weight loss make bad bedfellows. Let me count the ways. First, starting a meal off with a drink stimulates the appetite (that's why it's called an aperitif) and leads to eating more calories during the meal. Second, there are a substantial number of calories in adult beverages (with no other nutritional benefit), and the body doesn't hold up the "I'm full" stop sign any faster when you eat and drink simultaneously. Finally, alcohol messes with your mind's command and control center, so you tend to behave (and order and eat) more impulsively. In other words, the expression should be eat, drink, and be heavy.

# IN TRAINING FOR GAINING

The funny thing about my college weight gain is that it merely positioned me at normal weight for my height. In fact, I looked healthier, as I no longer looked like a hunger striker. If I could have applied the brakes right then, it would have been no problem, and I might not have been inspired to write this book. But I kept on gaining.

Between the ages of 21 and 25, I was launching my career,

working for a small consulting firm in Washington, DC. That meant working interminable hours for no money. But somehow I was expected to pay rent and make car payments. I had so little disposable income that I often resorted to ketchup and bread sandwiches for lunch. My only real splurge was paying the monthly fee at my local gym, where I turned up regularly, if at odd hours. I dropped to about 200 pounds, but I attribute it to the penniless postgrad diet.

In the fall of 1990, I made a big life change. I moved to Chicago to help a colleague open an office for the same small consulting firm, and I also enrolled in the Graduate School of Business at the University of Chicago. I began to find my groove and started to shed my childish ways. I got my MBA primarily by attending night classes, and this was as intense a period of work as I can remember. I also started dating Sandee, a friend from college and the woman who would soon become my wife. The Duke U Party Devil turned into something much more serious and did it while still working full-time.

After graduating from the University of Chicago, I was shocked to receive an offer to work for the Boston Consulting Group (BCG). To this day, I really do not understand why they gave me a job, as their usual pattern is to hire smart people who did not spend their undergraduate years majoring in frat-animal behavior. I was grateful for the chance to begin anew, so I threw myself into the job wholeheartedly, and my career started to move. But I also bade farewell to underweight, for good. To avoid blaming the real culprit (i.e., me), I blame two things: I was earning a decent paycheck, and I started to travel.

I love Chicago. In my 5 years there, I particularly learned to love the food—the deep-dish pizza and those high-piled Chicago hot dogs, inevitably served alongside an equally high-piled basket of cheese fries. Chicago is a dangerous place for a formerly food-deprived man-child with a brand-new credit card. All of a sudden, I could eat out anytime I wanted.

My diet in Chicago looked something like this.

**Breakfast:** A very large bowl of full-fat granola mixed with yogurt. What I find frightening is that I thought of this as the healthy part of my day. A serving size of granola is about 220 calories. Not so bad, right? That's 220 calories per ½ cup. I was easily eating two full cups of granola in that big bowl. That's nearly 900 calories, or almost half of the allotted calories for a guy my size to eat in a full day. I was in trouble before I'd even changed out of my pajamas.

**Lunch:** Wraps are healthy, right? Not when they're the size of my already plus-size forearm. My favorite was turkey slathered with mayo and filled with bacon, veggies, and other calorie bombs. In my nutritional pea brain, this was also a healthy meal because it was a wrap and it had turkey. Like a lot of people, I was giving myself credit for healthy ingredients while failing to factor in the stuff that went with it. Down the hatch!

**Dinner:** Hey, cut me a break. I'd already had (what I thought of as) two healthy meals! Now I opened my wallet and my mouth wide for Chinese, calzones, deep-dish pizza, BBQ, pasta with cream sauce—bring on the Alfredo, baby!

But wait, it gets worse. That was just the routine Monday through Friday. On weekends, I really cut loose. There were few things I loved more than rocking a monstrous breakfast. Giant omelets, four pieces of thick toast, home fries, bacon. Ahhhh. I don't need to calculate the nutritional consequences— they were all adding up around my waistline, belt notch by belt notch.

Of course, it just got worse because I was on the road two or three nights a week, comforting myself with food. As a kid, I never traveled much, and hotels were mysterious and beautiful places—gleaming buildings with comfortable rooms and a staff eager to wheel in carts of food from off the room service menu.

This was a dangerous place for a food hedonist like me. At one of my favorite hotels, I used to order quesadillas as a starter, and the serving could have fed a mariachi band. I'd follow that up with a club sandwich or a cheeseburger served with a pile of thick-cut fries. I scoured my plates clean, so I'd qualify for dessert. Have I mentioned that I have a thing for ice cream? Bring on the low-fat Ben & Jerry's, because that doesn't count, right?

People who successfully manage their weight often speak of the need to be in control—of their emotions, their environments, their schedules. Structure and routine make the job of self-monitoring (keeping track of exercise, food intake, and weight) easier. Change often challenges us to adjust the things we do to stay in control. When the change is physically or emotionally stressful, such as going to college, becoming a parent, or traveling for business (hey, I did all three!), the maintenance of desired lifestyle behaviors is further challenged. And that goes double in a hotel in Cleveland.

On the exercise front, I still tried to hit the gym, but I'd become truant, averaging seven to eight visits per month. I walked a lot with my wife, as Chicago is a wonderful walking city. But my caloric intake was far outpacing what I burned through walking and exercise. Midlife was truly settling in— around my belt line.

In retrospect, the fact that I gained another 30 pounds in my first few years at BCG was hardly a shock. I ate like an idiot. But if I dig deep for a moment, I admit there was more to it. At heart, I was a clean-plate-club guy just waiting for the opportunity for a hearty food binge, and I'd finally reached a point in my life where I could act out my hedonistic fantasies. I ate without thinking and gained without noticing . . . if I looked the other way when I walked past the bathroom mirror.

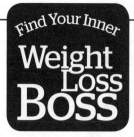

**You're surrounded by food enemies. Just don't bite them!**

## Note to self: It's *still* the environment, stupid!

Indisputably, the change in environment made my weight gain possible. I was surrounded by unlimited food everywhere I turned, from grocery stores to restaurants to hotels. With money in the bank and an expense account at my disposal, I now had the means to pillage my new food environment, and I was mentally and emotionally ill equipped to manage it. Our bodies are programmed to eat when the eating is good. My body was telling me to eat everything I could get my hands on, in case the Irish Potato Famine happened again. Multiply that by millions of people with similar instincts in our food-flush times, and you have a giant problem on your hands. But you can't burn every pizza joint to the ground. Instead, you need to find new pathways through that dangerous world to help you sidestep hazards and defuse calorie bombs.

## I'm not Superman, and neither are you.

I was hardly the first young guy to think I could do pretty much what I wanted without paying for it. I assumed that I was naturally skinny and would stay that way. I was uneducated about nutrition, and I was careless in the way that I ate. I deserved to gain weight because I took no responsibility for the decisions that I made around food. I would like to blame all of that on the industrial fast-food complex, but that's a cop-out. Yes, there are things that must change in our food environment, but the most important change had to be in myself.

There is no getting around the fact that if I was to start eating whatever I wanted whenever I wanted it, I would regain all of my weight and then some. I will always have to watch what I eat because I still live in the tempting food environment that got me heavy in the first place. I eventually came to realize that I had to respect that fact by taking steps to alter the way I interacted with my environment. Consider which environments cause you to lose your grip (buffets, say—or mindless eating at night). Simply being aware of these tendencies will help you get the upper hand.

# Weight Watchers Profile

## "You can do this. I know you can!"

How one man battled his obesogenic environment, and won

### Derrick Deaton, 28, *Westfield, IN*

**HEIGHT:** 6 feet 2 inches
**WEIGHT BEFORE:** 529
**WEIGHT AFTER:** 189
Reached his goal in 28 months

### MY STRUGGLE

My weight has been an issue my entire life. Growing up, I ate all the wrong foods—and too much of them. It's no surprise that I weighed 400 pounds by my senior year of high school, and by the time I was 26, I was taking two blood pressure medicines and suffered from severe sleep apnea. Even going to the grocery store had become arduous. My back would inevitably start hurting, forcing me to take breaks in the car. I was the biggest person everywhere I went. Stares, pointing, snickers—I experienced it all. My seat belt didn't fit. Every chair was my enemy. I couldn't sit in restaurant booths or go to any event that had stadium seating. Flying was terrible. My doctors were practically begging me to go under the knife for bariatric surgery.

### MY WAKE-UP CALL

My sister shed 50 pounds on Weight Watchers and was constantly asking me to sign up. Finally, one day, I caved and told her I would give it a week. When I walked into the center, I didn't think I'd be able to relate to anyone. I asked the meeting leader, Cyndi, "Have you seen anyone my size do this?" She looked right at me and said, "No, but the plan works, and if you stick with it, it will work for you." She smiled at me, took my arm, and said, "Derrick, you can do this! I know you can!" Something just clicked, and I knew I could do it. I haven't looked back since.

## MY FOOD

Before I lost the weight, I was a binge eater. I'd hit the drive-thru and order three or four sandwiches at a time. I could easily eat a whole medium pizza plus an order of breadsticks. And I never ate just one bowl of cereal—I'd have four. My biggest challenge was learning portion control. Now I eat a reasonably sized piece of grilled chicken for dinner, with carrots or green beans. It's hard, because fast food is cheap, and unhealthy options are everywhere. But I make sure never to shop hungry and don't allow myself to buy unhealthy foods, because I can't eat them if I don't have them. I always keep safe options on hand, while still allowing myself occasional treats. If I want my grandma's peanut butter pie, I simply make cuts elsewhere. The key to my success has been planning for it. I've completely changed the way I think about food.

## MY FITNESS

Incorporating exercise was hard. But I can proudly say I did it myself—I never had a trainer. I started small, with videos in my living room and walks around the neighborhood. I lost my first 220 pounds without ever setting foot in a gym. When I finally did join a gym, I started by walking on the treadmill and tried to set the speed a little higher each time. My weight loss doubled.

## MY PAYOFF

The way I'm treated now is so different. I was used to sticking out, and now I can blend in—in a good way. I grew up in a small town, and when I recently visited, people didn't recognize me. I was with my family, and friends kept asking, "Where's Derrick?" not realizing who I was. I never thought I'd be called skinny. But now I am. I owe my life to the plan.

# {CHAPTER 3}
# Man Meets Scale—
# Losing the Weight

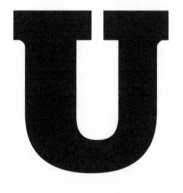**P TO NOW,** I've been going on at some length—and beating myself up—about the life progression that led to my maximum weight: 242 pounds at age 32. I'm telling this story for two reasons: (1) as a reminder to me that what happened once in my life could easily happen again, if I'm not vigilant; and (2) in hopes that you might identify with the food tsunami that washed over me and identify your own potential to fight back against the tide, just as I have.

It took me more than a decade to complete the transformation from skinny kid to big guy, and it took serious time for me to shed that weight as well. From my own journey back to a sensible weight, I know that the experience has its ups and downs. Since joining Weight Watchers in early 2000, I've met many members who have had wonderful success. Every time I meet a Lifetime Member (i.e., someone who has reached their ultimate goal weight), I hear a story that includes many twists, turns, starts, stops and restarts. It reinforces what I've come to know about weight loss: It's a hard job, and you've got to stick with it through good times and bad. But the payday is worth it and lasts a lifetime. Are you in?

If losing weight was simply a function of knowing what to do, the obesity epidemic would vanish within a year. However, downsizing is not so simple. The hard part is not just knowing what to do, it's being able to act on that knowledge and incorporate those changes into your life. Making it happen day to day, meal by meal, is where the real work is.

## My Basic Weight Loss Logic

• Losing weight sustainably requires establishing a healthy lifestyle.

• A healthy lifestyle is not a moral straitjacket. Rather, it is a combination of healthy habits you feel good about and can stick to.

• A habit is a behavior you execute without thinking. It could be waking up every weekday and going for a run, or it could be robotically munching potato chips while watching TV.

• The process of replacing unhealthy habits with healthy ones—running in the street, not to the cupboard for a bag of crunchy fat—is more involved than it seems.

You should take care to lose weight gradually and sensibly. Crash diets aren't any better than crash driving—they lead to negative results. But if you make steady progress, you're more likely to sustain those gains. A pound a week is plenty for the first several months. They really add up.

Most often, a weight loss attempt will be triggered by something—a New Year's resolution, the looming threat of swimsuit season, or the knowledge that people will be brandishing cameras or making judgments at a high school reunion or a wedding. Many say simply: "I do not want to live this way anymore. I need to deal with this issue now." That's why I've included the Weight Watchers Profiles at the end of every chapter. People tend to gain weight in similar ways, but every path to losing it is unique to the person who takes it. What will your way be?

Some combination of motivations pushed me to draw a line I never want to cross again. What follows is the story and timeline of my own weight loss, from the bad habits that weighed me down to the good ones that lifted me up. It was worth every day I spent.

# The Spark

I'm almost 33 years old, and the year is 1999. I had just moved to Connecticut to take a job working at PepsiCo in a corporate strategy group. I was making nearly weekly trips from New York to Bradenton, Florida, and I was starting to rack up some serious international miles. It was an exciting time, but it was also pretty intense.

On the home front, I had a 1-year-old daughter, Harley, so there were endless nights of interrupted sleep as well as the stress of being responsible for providing for a new life. My daughter had a ferocious case of colic, and she spent many hours of her first year furious at the world and not afraid to express herself fully and vocally.

This brew of travel, long hours, sleepless nights, and stress had a predictable outcome: I ate an awful lot of food. When I think back on it, I remember the nights sitting in hotel rooms, thankful for a couple of hours of peace in front of the TV. What else could I do but peruse the room service menu? It seems pretty obvious now that I was medicating my stress with food. Food was my reward, and I was convinced I deserved an epic one!

Having a tough day? Just wait until you get to your hotel room and dig into appetizers, burgers, and fries, followed by a dessert so big it had its own gravitational force. Have a few hours to relax on the weekend? Head out to the local grub pub to keep the "rewards" coming.

I continued to pile on weight. At this point, I avoided the scale; I didn't even know where our scale at home was. I would suck in my gut when I walked past mirrors and bought a wardrobe of loose-fitting clothes. I was deeply grateful to be living in an era when pleats were permissible.

Life continued like this until one day my wife started riding me about scheduling my annual checkup. I probably hadn't seen a doctor since business school, when university health services checked me out just to ensure that I didn't have a latent case of Ebola. My wife didn't say she was concerned about my weight, but she was wise enough to know that the doctor would bring it up. Grudgingly, I acquiesced to her loving pressure and set an appointment with a doctor in my little Connecticut town.

My physical completely sucked. Thanks, hon. The biggest pain came first, of course: the weigh-in. As I stepped up on the little platform, I felt as if I'd climbed onto the stage at Carnegie Hall without being able to sing. I kept telling myself that it couldn't be all that bad. My elements of denial—Turkey sandwiches! Low-fat ice cream! Road food doesn't count!—bubbled up as I looked hopefully toward a benign scale result. With one eye open.

I felt pretty sick as I watched the nurse manipulating the weights—sliding and scraping, sliding and scraping, from the land of the healthy into the heavyweight subdivision. It was like seeing my weight gain of the previous decade in time-lapse photography, settling far right on the scale and far beyond what was reasonable on my long frame. Oops, looks like we're going to need to move that 100-pound marker over one more time! It took an eternity for the scale pointer to reach its equilibrium.

The verdict: 242 pounds. Guilty as charged.

I felt the blood rush to my face. It was as if someone had given me a roundhouse straight to the gut, which the sweet

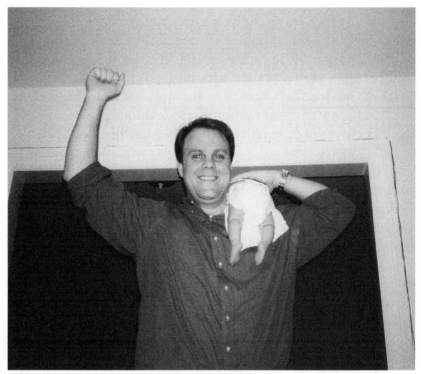

This is (a lot of) me in summer of 1998 with my newly minted daughter Harley. Would someone please help this man?!

blameless nurse certainly had. For someone who had been thin to the point of emaciation for the first two decades of his life, 240 was a freaking huge number. I was furious—at myself, at the world that had tempted me with too much food. Was I past the point of no return?

But the scary experiences and humiliations just kept coming. One week later, I returned to the doctor's office for a review of my blood work. My cholesterol clocked in at 260: HDL 50 (approaching high), LDL 181 (high). My doctor told me I should probably start on a regimen of statins (i.e., Lipitor) to bring down my already too-high cholesterol levels as I was pretty far out of the range. In a nutshell, she told me I was well on my way to having the chronic diseases that kill most Americans. She also wanted me to get my weight under control: My BMI was a 30, which indicated that I was clinically obese. She then ran a quick calculation on the number of calories I should be eating per day in order to lose the weight over a period of time: around 1,800, aka my favorite Marriott quesadilla "appetizer." Not only would losing weight be good for my cholesterol numbers and blood pressure, it would help reduce my risk of other dreaded diseases, such as type 2 diabetes.

At this point, the physical was over and the deep-seated panic began.

Wait a minute! High cholesterol? Clinical obesity? Me? I'm only 32 years old! Statins are for people my dad's age! Obesity is for . . . fat people!

Like me. The answer for me was either to take a lot of new drugs to fight a bad health prognosis or to change the way I lived in order to live longer and healthier.

In my current line of work, I've met many people whose weight problems and related health conditions were at least as bad, if not worse. I think I know exactly how each of them must have felt when they first received the cold slap of truth from a nurse or doctor. For me, this was the moment when I could no longer deny that my weight problem demanded immediate action. I could no longer fall back on my usual evasions: "I look fine!" "I'm a big guy, and it's okay to weigh this much!"

Now I knew those were lies. I had to do something! But what?

# Caught in a Fat Trap

As soon as I got home, I confessed my failings to my wife. I swore at myself and uttered other terms of self-loathing and reproach. She was sympathetic, of course, but I also got the feeling that she was glad the doctor had leveled with me. She promptly walked over to the bookshelf and gave me a paperback book filled with the caloric values of different foods. It was time for me to start counting calories.

That night, I pulled out a notepad and started recording the calories of everything I ate that day. I felt like I was finally doing something, rather than just silently worrying. Yay me! Go David! I went to sleep that night with the feeling that this whole problem would be a distant memory in just a few months. I was entering my new life of responsibility and propriety!

For the next few days, I kept track of my calories, more or less, and I found myself becoming more aware of my food choices. I started to make a number of food switches, going for the Baked! Lay's instead of the high-test variety. I earnestly tried to make better decisions as I walked through the cafeteria at work, filled with a sense of personal responsibility. (But it was PepsiCo, after all.)

What happened next was fairly predictable. I fell into the same trap that has ensnared so many others. Within about 10 days, I stopped counting calories altogether. My reason: I felt that I was already making better decisions and that I had figured it out. I was now a responsible member of society, and I did not need my calorie book any longer. It had served its purpose.

If only it were that easy, right?

In the weeks that followed, I kept on behaving responsibly. Really. But I can see now that I started to unconsciously make fewer good choices and more bad ones. My excuse-making mechanisms kicked in again, and I told myself that some of my choices were not really so bad. I remained ignorant of my portion sizes, guesstimating badly and with abandon. I slipped back into my old life, but with healthy living as window dressing. The house behind it was as big as ever: The weight I lost initially came back, and I found myself knocking on the door of 240 again.

In hindsight, I see that my first stabs at weight loss never had a chance. I never gave my new healthy practices enough

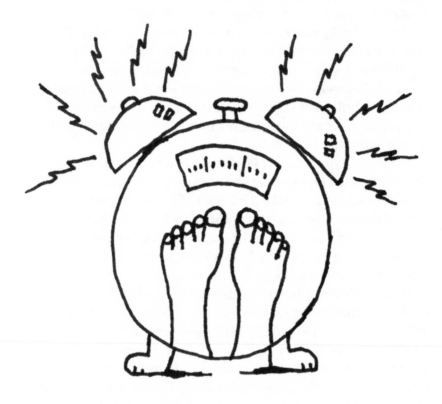

time to actually become ingrained as habits. I wasn't learning to be more mindful about how and when I was actually eating. I wasn't really being systematic about my food choices. I still didn't know what a proper portion was, and I didn't really want to know.

I was simply learning to rationalize in a new way. I would order the bran muffin instead of the blueberry muffin, never mind the fact that there was no real nutritional difference between them. One seemed "healthier," and that was good enough. So my "new patterns" were just another take on the same old patterns that had caused the problem in the first place. I needed a process, and I needed mechanisms to keep me engaged and focused.

# MY FIRST WEIGHT WATCHERS MEETING

It is now late January 2000. I have left PepsiCo to take a job at an Internet start-up, WeightWatchers.com, Inc., as employee number six. We had survived Y2K without losing our dial tone, though we were left with an awful lot of bottled water and batteries in our basement. I was a fully portly guy again, having enjoyed—thoroughly—another holiday eatathon.

By way of background, Weight Watchers was sold by Heinz in late 1999 in a leveraged buyout led by its management and Artal, a European investment group advised by the Invus Group. For the first time since the late 1970s, Weight Watchers International was again its own company, not beholden to another corporate keeper. It was an exciting time, full of possibilities, and one of them was the Internet.

In 1999, the Internet was run by rooms full of monkeys at keyboards, with a flurry of business plans being generated every day. Down was up, initial public offerings were making people rich, and nobody recognized that this was the Dutch tulip mania of 1637 all over again. Sure enough, there were dozens of Internet start-ups popping up, focusing on online dieting. This created both an opportunity and a challenge for Weight Watchers, which was traditionally very much a face-to-face, "high touch" company made up of lots of caring people. We were great with people, but, with little to no technological aptitude, we were not so great with the person-machine interface.

The management team at Weight Watchers International was completely swamped with new initiatives, including getting on as an independent company and launching our revolutionary Points program. At the time, the Weight Watchers Web site was probably about eight pages deep, carrying fascinating stuff like listings of meeting locations. Weight Watchers management feared that if the Internet remained a pet project buried within its organization, our

Web site would never have the focus to allow it to realize its potential. In partnership with its board, WeightWatchers. com, Inc. was created as a stand-alone, independent company in late 1999.

Like a lot of type A guys my age, I had dreams of joining a start-up while I was toiling away in corporate anonymity at PepsiCo. I remember very clearly the day that a friend called me up to tell me that he was thinking about taking the business development/marketing/strategy role at the newly formed WeightWatchers.com. He wanted to brainstorm about the opportunity. My reaction at the time was: huh? Back then, I thought Weight Watchers was a frozen food company, and the notion of creating a start-up to peddle frozen food seemed like kind of a dumb idea. My friend patiently explained that Weight Watchers was actually an education and behavior-change program. He explained its new system called Points, which assigned each individual a target number to reach each day, based on the caloric values of the foods that person was eating. The idea was to help people manage food intake through budgeting and tracking the calories in the foods they ate.

My friend and I continued to brainstorm about this new concept during those weeks in December 1999. My wife had always been an avid user of Quicken to manage the family financials, and I started to wonder if Weight Watchers could develop something similar online. I passed on these ideas to my friend, but then one day he called to tell me he wasn't going to take the job. He couldn't justify moving his family up to New York from DC. He asked if I would be interested in talking to the investors about joining in his place. My response? Yes!

I was one of the first senior hires at this new start-up, starry-eyed with dreams of being part of a fabulously successful Internet company that would certainly be worth bajillions of dollars in no time. My bubble, and the Internet's, burst on April 4, 2000, thereby ending the era of brainless Internet millions.

I wouldn't be able to buy the New York Knicks after all. But really, I was fine with the new world order. I knew we were building a real business. If our products actually helped people lose weight, they would pay for them. On this basis, we relied on a subscription-based program despite the popular belief at the time that this model would be unsustainable.

On my first day at work, I walked into our ramshackle office space in lower midtown Manhattan—part online operation, part Weight Watchers print magazine. I sat at my desk, and I realized that I had no idea where to start. So much for the glamour of a start-up. First, I needed to figure out what Weight Watchers actually did.

It was time to start going to meetings. The people I'd meet there could be my focus group, and maybe I could start losing some weight. I found a meeting at a nearby synagogue on 36th Street, and I remember very clearly walking up to the door with my stomach lodged against my esophagus. This was an alien environment, and I had no idea what to expect.

I walked through the doors to see a group of women in a large open room with rows of folding chairs. In the back of the room was a long table with three women busily handling paperwork and weighing in the attendees. At this point, I was not yet a member of the program, and I did not announce myself as a Weight Watchers employee. What would they have thought, given the way I looked at the time? It wasn't the last time I measured my image against my company's promises.

I was completely lost in this female-dominated haven for the formerly heavy, but I filled out a registration form, paid my $12, and was weighed in. I was given a membership book along with a bunch of materials to help me launch my own weight loss regimen.

Ironically, my first leader was, of all things, a guy. Michael Filan is a classic New Yorker who spends part of his time doing management coaching, part of it working as a Weight Watchers leader, and part of it as an artist. I listened to him talk about his own weight loss experience, and I sat rapt as other members shared their experiences. At the end of the meeting, there was a Getting Started session where Michael walked new members through the program.

So what happened during that daunting first hour? What did I learn? In truth, I was not a typical new member in that I had now been working for WeightWatchers.com for a few weeks. I had read a lot of the materials even before I had taken the job. Learning about the program and how it worked was one of the reasons I wanted to join the company in the first place. That said, I had a couple of big impact moments during that very first Weight Watchers meeting.

# WEIGHT LOSS MADE SIMPLE

### ONE: It's pretty much common sense

It's funny, but when I was learning about Weight Watchers on my own, I think I had overcomplicated it in my head (I have a gift for doing this). When I sat down for my 15-minute Getting Started session, Michael took me through a drill that made the whole process seem fairly basic.

In a nutshell, each person is allocated a budget of Points per day. Every food has a Points value, and all you have to do is stay within your budget. I learned how to calculate a Points value, which back then was based on a combination of calories, fat (bad), and fiber (good) using a paper slide rule. Further, Michael walked me through the process of using a paper tracker to keep score each day (imagine your checkbook record), as these were still olden times, before all of our fancy new Internet and mobile applications. I also learned that I could win Points values back by doing a bunch of exercise (they call these Activity Points). Michael went on to talk about all of the different ways I could get support and help, as well as the importance of attending my meeting each week to help me stay on track. This wasn't nearly as complicated as I thought it was going to be.

In truth, there is a lot more to the Weight Watchers program than what I just listed above, but this is really all you need to know following your first meeting or experience. At its core, the program is pretty simple; its richness comes in everything you learn about a lean lifestyle, along with tools to affect longer term changes in how you live your life. More on that later.

## **TWO:** I was now standing on the precipice of changing my life

I will admit that it felt weird to start an actual weight loss process using a real-life, officially designated program, as opposed to my previous, largely improvised weight loss attempts. But this was kind of exciting because I could finally visualize losing my weight in a way that felt logical to me. It also completely freaked me out, because I was finally admitting to myself, in a public place, that I needed help to deal with my weight. I finally acknowledged that my weight problem was bigger than me, and I needed to reach outside my own resources to conquer it. This was no small statement.

In truth, the weirdness of being a guy on Weight Watchers dissipated pretty quickly. Attending meetings, reckoning Points, and exercising were just things I was doing to lose weight. The alien-ness of it all lasted less than a day. The harder part for me: What to do first? How about after that? What was I supposed to eat? What's for dinner? Would anybody want to eat lunch with me? How many Points values are there in . . . everything? I was engaged in the most basic process there is: figuring out how to retool my whole life through better choices.

I walked out of my first meeting, stood on Lexington Avenue, and thought to myself: "I, David Kirchhoff, am now a Weight Watchers member." Not exactly where I saw my life headed when I was younger.

# STICKING WITH THE PROGRAM, AND LOSING

For the next week, I dutifully wrote down everything I ate all day and calculated the Points values. (I couldn't track it on Weight Watchers Online then, as I can now, because I hadn't launched it yet.) The first few days were a little painful. The shift from eating a truckload of food each day to eating about 1,700 calories was pretty radical. Afternoons, I developed a hunger headache, and by dinner I was pretty antsy. It was like delirium tremens, but for a foodaholic. Looking back, I was probably a little overzealous in my efforts (that type A problem again) and hadn't really been paying attention to Michael's pointers on how to avoid feelings of hunger and deprivation during that first week.

At my next meeting, I was eager to hop on the scale. I had worked hard over the past 7 days, and, dammit, I wanted a result to show for it. If memory serves, I lost about 5 pounds my first week. Go, Dave! (You've got to love that water weight loss during the first week or two.)

The second week, the headaches went away and I started to feel normal on my new regimen. I quickly learned to renavigate my local environment, and I found some meals at the neighborhood Au Bon Pain that were very much on plan. I was suddenly living the life of food chastity. My puritan forbearers would have been proud!

More important, I had one of my first major epiphanies since taking the job at Weight Watchers. At a local New York meeting, the leader called attention to a member who had recently reached her 100-pound weight loss milestone. This wonderful young woman had spent the prior 2 years transforming her life in an amazing and fundamental way. I was astonished and inspired. I was proud to be rid of my 5 pounds, and she'd worked through twenty times that. Where did she find the strength? That's when I realized that the organization I had joined was far more than an ordinary business. This was the day I drank the Weight Watchers Kool-Aid—a metaphor that is wrong on too many levels to list them all.

Inspired by her story and my own evident need, I lost about 25 pounds in the next few months. I was converted. I could not remember the last time I had weighed as little as 215, and I was pretty proud. I was also beginning to lift weights a couple of times per week, and I began to incorporate good stuff like fruit into my diet. Just as negative momentum had overcome me in my midtwenties, I started gaining speed in a new, positive direction. I felt better physically, and I frankly liked the way I looked. My pants were suddenly starting to feel loose, and I had to overtighten my belt to prevent a wardrobe malfunction. It was bad fashion, but a really good sign about where I was headed in life.

At this point, my days as a 240-pound guy seemed pretty firmly behind me. I got a grip on the basics of living healthier, and I was much less prone to the food crimes of my past life. Chinese food was a distant memory, and my calzone habit went away. We were cooking healthier at home, and I was starting to feel comfortable in my new life.

I even spent a weekend attending Basic Leader Skills, the introductory training course for all new Weight Watchers leaders. Every single one of my fellow classmates had lost weight and kept it off on the program, so I was in great company. I spent two days with a fabulous cadre of people, learning to run meetings, facilitate discussions among members, and celebrate their success. I was becoming a true believer.

So that was it, right? Having done the program this one time, could I now call myself cured?

Sadly, no.

# Kirchhoff:
# The Missing (7) Years

As noted, weight loss is often not a direct journey. It has its twists and turns, ups and downs. There are periods where you are highly focused and times when you wear doughnut glasses. This was certainly the case with me.

During this long interval, my weight fluctuated from a high of 225 to a low of typically 215, depending on what was happening in my life (and my stomach). I'd made a lot of progress from where I started, but I hadn't reached my destination of peace and leanness—not by a long stretch.

One of the strengths of Weight Watchers is that the coaches quickly identify—and encourage the pursuit of—two key weight loss milestones: 10 percent and Lifetime Membership. Ten percent is simply realizing that much loss from the starting weight. Of course, there's nothing simple about it. You receive a key chain for achieving this milestone, but more important, you receive the benefit of having significantly reduced your future health risk factors, particularly diabetes.

Achieving Lifetime Membership is a little more complicated. You qualify for this one when you reach your goal weight (typically when your BMI is 25) and hold it—plus or minus 2 pounds—for 6 weeks. Why the 6 weeks? After losing weight, you need to learn how to hold it steady. How to eat a bit more so as to stop losing but not so much as to begin regaining. It takes a while to get the hang of this (both mentally and physically). By continuing weekly contact with Weight Watchers after hitting your ultimate weight goal, you've got the support to help you make the transition.

Once you achieve Lifetime Membership at Weight Watchers, you can attend meetings for free forever as long as you are within 2 pounds of that goal weight and you weigh in at least once per month. It's a pretty big deal for Weight Watchers members. It does not happen for most, and it does not need to happen for most. However, it's a pretty special achievement and a definite badge of courage.

At my new weight level, I was within a few pounds of reaching my 10 percent milestone, but I never quite got there. Further, I was many more pounds from achieving Lifetime Membership. For some reason, I just couldn't keep it together long enough to hit these two marks.

For some reason? Actually, I wasn't able to hit these marks for easily identifiable reasons: Even working for the company, drinking the Kool-Aid, selling the program to others, and seeing the results it could achieve, I was not yet fully committed to living a healthier life.

During these lost 7 years, my list of not very good habits was just too long to overcome with periodic bursts of good intentions. For example, I was still making stupid lunch mistakes. Every time I put the tracker away and start trusting my instincts, I got into trouble. I fell back on the trick of looking at the window dressing of a food and guesstimating its nutritional content. One day, I pulled the nutritional information from the Web site of a local lunch place, and I found that the wraps I assumed to be healthy were twice the calories I'd guessed—and therefore likely to settle in for a long stay on my waistline. Yogurt parfaits that I was treating as a little side with those wraps were almost as bad. I was eating nearly 75 percent of my daily caloric allotment at lunch, which didn't leave much margin for breakfast and dinner. I was self-sabotaging through arrogance: I believed I knew what to eat, but I was far from being an expert.

Travel continued to trip me up. Out of town, out of mind, evidently. I convinced myself that if food happened in my room, it wouldn't follow me out the door when I checked out. Even with my Weight Watchers training, I would still order the American Breakfast for room service—that's a euphemism for one of everything (e.g., eggs, toast, meat, pastries, Hansel and Gretel, etc.). My weekends were Weight Watchers–free because, hey, it was the weekend!

Throughout these years, I would cycle from being super-diligent to being pretty lax. It was amazing: My weight would follow suit! Each time I would gain, I would move on to self-loathing, pull on my hair shirt, and enter a phase of extreme discipline and painful deprivation. Nor did I enjoy the feeding frenzies, because I felt out of control. Basically, I was yo-yo dieting.

There. I admitted it. For many of my first 7 years on Weight Watchers, I was treating it like a diet. When I use the word *diet,* I am usually using it in a very specific way—an unnatural eating regimen undertaken for 2 to 3 months before returning to life as usual.

For too many years, I would use the mechanics of the Weight Watchers food plan to "fix" a temporary weight problem, but I was not truly dealing with my underlying problems and challenges. This was only sinning against myself, but it was holding me back nonetheless.

I needed a new spark to push it all the way.

# My Second Spark
## (And I May Need a Third, One Day)

If you had asked me when I was 20 years old if I ever thought I would end up being the CEO of Weight Watchers, I would have asked you the following questions:

"What is Weight Watchers?"

"Have you mistaken me for a woman?"

Not that the "woman" part of the company bothered me. When I first started working for Weight Watchers, I simply thought of my part of the company as an Internet start-up that happened to serve women. During the next 7 years, the roles I had were mostly in the context of the Internet business, and they generally were financial and strategy roles. I did not begin to see myself fully as a leader in the organization until I became CEO of WeightWatchers.com in 2004. Even then, the Web operations were still a separate company. It was not until I really started to live the Weight Watchers life that I began to appreciate the role and mission of the company.

A sequence of events starting in the summer of 2005 began to change everything for me. In July of that year, the company I helped start was acquired and became a fully majority-subsidiary of Weight Watchers International. I was still the CEO of WeightWatchers.com, but I was now reporting to the CEO of Weight Watchers International, Linda Huett. About 2 months after the acquisition, Linda asked me to take on the additional responsibility of overseeing the traditional meetings business outside of North America. I now had two jobs, COO of International Operations and CEO of WeightWatchers.com. I went about this new role of living Weight Watchers in 20-plus countries outside the United States for the next 12 months, and my nose was pressed firmly to the grindstone.

One year into this role, I learned that Linda, my mentor of the past 7 years, was planning to announce her retirement as CEO. In what I can only describe as a desperate move, the board asked me to be her internal successor. Why do I say desperate? Simple: Linda was and is an absolute force of nature. How could I possibly fill her shoes?

Linda is a product of the Yale Drama School and a former actress who met a Brit and soon found herself married with children in London. After 10 years in business, Linda had three kids over the span of 18 months and had gained 70 pounds, and who could blame her? She was able to lose 30 on her own, but she realized that she needed help to nail the last 40. She joined Weight Watchers on her twins' first birthday, and within a year she was back to her pre-childbirth weight. She then became a Weight Watchers leader in the United Kingdom. From there, Linda held just about every management job you could have in that operation, including VP and managing director. Linda and her team designed the original Points system. When Artal acquired Weight Watchers from Heinz in 1999, the new board asked Linda to become CEO. She took the company public in 2001 and grew it from a roughly $300 million revenue company to one with more than $1 billion in sales.

In some sense, Linda *was* Weight Watchers. She had progressed from frontline leader to CEO. She knew every detail of the business intimately. She is a brilliant and intensely passionate woman who lived and breathed Weight Watchers. Her instincts for how to serve members were born out of her own personal experience, and every inch of the business felt her presence.

And then I came along.

Replacing (fat chance) this beloved figure was (1) a guy, (2) a guy with an MBA, and (3) a guy with an MBA who couldn't even reach goal weight, even without balancing twins and a toddler. Don't get me wrong. I brought skills and capabilities to the job, but as far as the beating heart of the business, how could I ever hope to know it as well as Linda did?

I spent the next 12 months conducting town hall meetings with staff around the United States and abroad. To get to know the basics of the business, I took training as a meeting receptionist, the person who checks members in for the crucial weigh-in. The first time I had to weigh someone in was a terrifying experience. More terrifying still was the first time I had to weigh someone in who had gained weight that week. Perhaps more personally significant, this also became the spark that ultimately got me to my goal weight.

# BETTING ON ME

It is now early 2007, and I had been CEO for about 3 months. We had just made a decision to up the ante at our NYC headquarters and encourage everyone there to fully embrace living on the program. We sponsored a charity drive based on weight loss achieved at our weekly At Work meeting at our head office. I corralled a few of my colleagues to create our own little weight loss competition—slapping a wager on our ability to stick with the Weight Watchers program and show results.

The bet was a fairly familiar one. Five of us set the goal of losing 10 percent of our body weight in the next 3 months. Everyone ponied up $100. If you reached your goal, you got your money back. If you failed, your money was split by everyone who succeeded. Let the trash-talking begin.

Everyone had made pretty good progress. I fought my weight down to 210 pounds, a new low in my own recent history. I had never looked or felt better. It turns out that this jolt was what I needed to make the finish line.

Using competition and incentives to spur weight loss is an intense area of research. The results have been mixed, especially relating to maintenance of the weight loss after the competition has ended. Also, it's important to structure contests so they focus on losing weight in a healthy way and at a safe and sustainable rate. That way, you can keep on moving once you pass the finish line.

Over the next couple of years, my weight gradually dropped, with minor ups and downs, from 210 in mid-2007 to the low 200s by the end of 2008. In early 2009, in consultation with my leader, Liz Josefsberg, and our chief science officer, Karen Miller-Kovach, I made the decision to set my goal weight at 203. In March 2009, I made it.

Took long enough!

One of the reasons I like to share this story is because it's a pretty good reflection of the reality of weight management. Changing behavior is not like changing a lightbulb. Establishing habits takes time, and often the right set of circumstances have to be in place to achieve real breakthroughs. I had to work at it for a long time. I suspect I will always have to work at. It's never a straight line, or at least it hasn't been for me. If I had expected my weight loss to work perfectly the first time, I would have been disappointed and probably quit the program. Next step: back at 240 or worse. In other words, realism, persistence, and patience are key ingredients to making it through to the other side. So is forgiveness. None of us are perfect, but we can triumph over imperfection if we know that and still strive to be better.

# Behavior Change and You

There is a time-tested psychological model for behavior change used to overcome a variety of conditions, from smoking to obesity. It's called the Prochaska model, named for a professor of psychology at the University of Rhode Island who pioneered the research, and it suggests that people have to go through a series of steps as they try to change their behavior. They are:

**Precontemplation:** "People are not intending to take action in the foreseeable future, and are most likely unaware that their behavior is problematic."

**Contemplation:** "People are beginning to recognize that their behavior is problematic, and start to look at the pros and cons of their continued actions."

**Planning:** "People are intending to take action in the immediate future, and may begin taking small steps towards change."

**Action:** "People have made specific overt modifications in their lifestyle, and positive change has occurred."

**Maintenance:** "People are working to prevent relapse, a stage which can last indefinitely."

**Termination:** "Individuals have zero temptation and 100% self-efficacy . . . they are sure they will not return to their old unhealthy habit as a way of coping."

Here's how my own warped mind translated these stages into action in my life:

**Precontemplation:** I'm tall and big. I look just fine. Now step away from my not-yet-finished enormous burrito before I chew your arm off.

**Contemplation:** Ooops. I'm a lot heavier than I thought I was, and this is not a good thing. It makes me sad when my doctor shakes his head that way.

**Planning:** Is there some sort of book I can read to make this go away? I really need to find a way to deal with this.

**Action:** I've now walked into my first Weight Watchers meeting, I'm now tracking Points values, and I'm taking my weigh-ins like a man.

**Maintenance:** I'm definitely skinnier, but I'm pretty sure that I'm at serious risk of regaining every single pound back and then some. I need to keep my game face on (and not stuff it too often).

**Termination:** I'll never get there. I will always be in maintenance, and that's okay with me. It energizes me to be fighting the good fight.

Years ago, Karen Miller-Kovach oversaw a really interesting piece of internal research at Weight Watchers. She wanted to understand the common elements among people who had repeatedly tried to lose weight. Some of their attempts were failures; others worked well. What she learned was exceedingly simple. Those who lost weight shared two common attributes.

- **They had a sense of urgency.** Losing weight wasn't just "important," it was more important than other priorities. Lifestyle change took precedence over—or fit into—the rest of the demands on their time.

- **They believed both in themselves and in their ability to comply with the weight loss approach they had chosen.** They knew that if they simply followed the program and stuck with it, it would work over time. This was in contrast to people who were convinced that they would most likely fail but felt that they owed it to themselves to try.

Karen's research parallels what other researchers have found—that being in a "good place" in one's life and believing in one's ability to do what is asked (called self-efficacy) are far more important than motivation and willpower in achieving weight loss success.

As CEO of Weight Watchers, and as a guy who has been on the program and succeeded, then failed, then succeeded some more, I can tell you this: You have what it takes to lose weight. You just need some tools to help you succeed.

You've come to the right place.

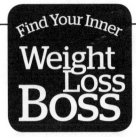

# The scale is like an honest friend: It never lies. Here is how to make it show winning numbers.

## Make it matter

For myself, I really did need the spark that would make dealing with my weight issue a top-5 priority in my life. In my case, it was a doctor completely freaking me out, and later, it was getting this job. I have met so many people who have lost a lot of weight, and they all have different sparks. What they share, though, is that losing the weight really mattered and therefore became a priority. Ask yourself why you really want to deal with your weight issue. Ask yourself if you believe weight loss will have a meaningful impact on the quality of your life. Do it for the right reasons, but find the right reasons to do it.

## Go into your weight loss effort with confidence

If you tell yourself that you will probably fail or bounce back to your old weight, then that's pretty much what will happen. On the other hand, if you go into this process with a belief that you can and want to live in a different, healthier, and more fulfilling way, you have a real shot. If you further remind yourself that you are fully capable of changing how you interact with food and exercise, then you can absolutely succeed. I have met so many people with so many different personalities and circumstances who succeeded. People are always stronger than they give themselves credit for. Give yourself credit, have faith, and have confidence.

## But also, learn to manage your expectations

Again, it took me 9 years to finally reach my goal weight. Adopting a healthy lifestyle is not a straight path. It is a winding path with steep ups and downs. The biggest mistake you can make is to give up on yourself after a big fall. Further, you should expect that you will periodically fall—I did it so often I'm surprised I can still walk. Haven't lost weight in a few weeks? Stay calm. Analyze what you've been doing. Make some changes in what you are doing. But do not quit! Stay with it, return to it, and you will eventually find your groove.

# Weight Watchers Profile

## "Now I eat to live, I don't live to eat."

A doctor's visit created urgency—and accountability

**Edwin Hood, 35,** *Garland, TX*

**HEIGHT:** 5 feet 10 inches
**WEIGHT BEFORE:** 356
**WEIGHT AFTER:** 245
Reached his goal in 87 weeks

### MY STRUGGLE

When I was growing up along the Jersey Shore, my weight controlled my life. At amusement parks, I couldn't fit on roller coasters. At the beach, I was too embarrassed to take my shirt off. On an airplane, I had to request a seat-belt extension. I sacrificed things so people wouldn't stare at me or so I wouldn't be the brunt of the jokes. I always thought dieting was for women. I just figured I'd always be big.

### MY WAKE-UP CALL

My family used to always say I was going to get diabetes, high cholesterol and high blood pressure. So whenever I had a doctor's appointment, I felt anxious that the doctor would find something. I knew that if I was ever going to lose weight it had to be now. I thought, "If I don't do something, all of these things I'm afraid of having are going to happen to me."

### MY FOOD

Before, I ate fast-food breakfast sandwiches, fries, doughnuts and a mocha drink—and that was just for breakfast. During the day, I'd snack on candy bars and chips and grab fast food for lunch. For dinner, I sometimes ate an entire small pizza. There was no feeling. I was just eating out of habit. Now I eat to live, I don't live to eat. I'm trying to provide fuel for my body to keep me going. I snack on fruits and vegetables and eat chicken with rice and greens on the side. I can't even eat fast food anymore without getting sick!

## MY FITNESS

I was too fat to run on the high school track team. Now I'm training for a half-marathon. I love taking group fitness classes—like spinning—at the gym. Once I finish spinning, I'll run a mile or two. At first it was intimidating to go into the gym and see all of the muscular guys. But now I'm the person in the front of the class telling people to stay with it.

## MY PAYOFF

I got my life back and I never knew it was lost. In high school, it took me 15 to 20 minutes to walk a mile. Now I'm running 8- to 10-minute miles. Weight Watchers didn't deprive me of anything. It held me accountable for who I truly am. A lot of guys look at dieting as a girl thing. But this process really just reprograms the way you think. Taking back control of your life? That's manly.

# PART II
# Be the Boss of Your Own Weight Loss:
Food, Tools, and Strategies to Take Charge for Life

# {CHAPTER 4}

# How to Make Food Your Friend—

## And Banish Deprivation

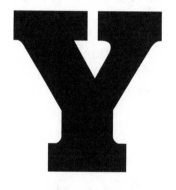**OU CAN'T WRITE A BOOK ABOUT LOSING WEIGHT** (and keeping it off) without a good, robust discussion of food. Calorically speaking, food is the component that largely determines whether we are gaining or losing weight. It all comes down to the kinds of foods we eat and the amounts of them we consume.

In more than a decade with Weight Watchers—as an employee and a member—I've gleaned a tremendous amount of knowledge about food. No, I'm not a nutritionist, but I have learned by attending Weight Watchers meetings, by listening to the people who work at my company, and by trying to stay current on research.

What follows is not intended to be a substitute for what one might learn from the expert sources at Weight Watchers or from a licensed nutritionist. But all of us would agree that we need to focus on food choices we can live with forever.

If there is one single point to take away from the following discussion on food, it is this: Please do not live in deprivation. If you are constantly hungry, you will fall back on your old choices. You can handle being hungry for a few days or weeks or even possibly a couple of months. But at some point, you will give in and throw the whole process out the window. Rather, the key is to choose foods that make you happy, keep you full, fit into your life, and are great calorie and nutrition bargains.

I really don't focus on the micronutrients in the foods I eat. I assume that if I eat enough quality foods (i.e., vegetables, fruits, fish, etc.), then my antioxidants and omega-3s will take care of themselves. But I do think a lot about foods that make me feel like I'm cheating the devil. These foods look huge, taste great, keep me full, and yet have few calories. They are the reason I've been at my goal weight for a good 3 years, and I never run around hungry.

In this chapter, I'll use my own best picks to illuminate the points I want to make. I may be a dietary exhibitionist, but I'm doing it for your benefit. You will have to find your own happy food Nirvana, but know this: It is there and waiting for you. You simply need to discover it.

# THE BASICS:
## What You Really Need to Know about Food

Wander around any Barnes & Noble, and you will find a whole section of the store dedicated to books about what you should eat. It can feel a little overwhelming. Here's the good news: Healthy eating is actually pretty simple!

I'm always amazed by the food fight surrounding certain nutritional topics—carbs versus protein versus fat, for instance. I have seen researchers on discussion panels nearly come to blows over fine distinctions between macronutrient interactions and hormone secretion (ick). I don't begrudge them their search for understanding, but for most of us, their debates are of limited use. In truth, most of us eat so poorly that merely becoming more mindful of what we eat would be a huge step in a smaller direction.

For all their battles, nutrition experts inevitably agree on the basic foods we should eat. Heart health diet pioneer Dean Ornish, MD, and Arthur Agatston, MD (*The South Beach Diet*), would seem to live in different universes, yet their ultimate recommendations on food are more alike than different. Eat fruits, vegetables, lean proteins, whole grains and low-fat dairy. So is there a last word on this subject so that we can all agree and move on to trickier topics?

The US government has recently taken a stab at providing just that. Every 5 years, the Department of Health and Human Services and the U.S. Department of Agriculture jointly publish the *Dietary Guidelines for Americans*.

To produce the *Dietary Guidelines,* lots of very knowledgeable people combed through mountains of scientific studies to answer roughly 180 questions related to the way we should eat. The results can be found on the USDA's Web site (www.cnpp.usda.gov/dietaryguidelines.htm). It is actually a pretty easy and interesting read, all collected and collated in the interest of making you over in the image of Uncle Sam (lean and vigorous), rather than leaving you to look like our recent budget deficits (round and red).

So what's in the new *Dietary Guidelines*? Mostly common sense, and that is a welcome addition to the usual nonsense about food.

# THE NEW DIETARY GUIDELINES, IN TWO (OKAY, FIVE) SENTENCES

- **Maintain calorie balance over time to achieve and sustain a healthy weight.** Translation: Don't eat too much and work plenty of activity into your life to lose weight and sustain the losses.

**• Focus on consuming nutrient-dense foods and beverages.** Translation: Eat more food that is high in nutrients and low in calorie density. Translation of translation: Eat mostly food that's good for you.

If that last bit seems a little vague, you are probably not alone in thinking that. There's plenty of confusion out there over what *good* means, what with food labels screaming largely meaningless health claims like "low fat," "natural," "multigrain," and "cholesterol-free food." Here's one way to cut through that marketingspeak: Buy foods that don't have labels! That is, shop for fruits, vegetables, dairy, and meat— each in their purest and least adulterated state—and you'll be in pretty good shape before you know it.

The *Dietary Guidelines* recommend that we limit sodium and foods with added sugars and fats (i.e., junk food). But I was most interested in the foods they want us to focus on. Here are their recommendations:

• Increase vegetable and fruit intake.

• Eat a variety of vegetables—especially dark-green, red, and orange ones—beans, and peas.

• Consume at least half of all grains as whole grains. Increase whole grain intake by replacing refined grains with whole grains.

• Increase intake of fat-free or low-fat milk and milk products, such as milk, yogurt, cheese, or fortified soy beverages.

• Choose a variety of protein foods, which include seafood, lean meat and poultry, eggs, beans, peas, soy products, and unsalted nuts and seeds.

• Increase the amount and variety of seafood consumed by choosing seafood in place of some meat and poultry.

• Replace protein foods that are higher in solid fats with choices that are lower in solid fats and calories and/or are sources of healthy oils.

• Use oils to replace solid fats where possible.

• Choose foods that provide more potassium, dietary fiber, calcium, and vitamin D, which are nutrients of concern in American diets. These foods include vegetables, fruits, whole grains, and milk and milk products.

You're right. Nobody will be able to remember all that. So the government came up with a simple mnemonic: a dinner plate. Fill half with fruits and vegetables, a quarter with whole grains, and a quarter with protein. Dairy is represented by a glass of low-fat milk, next to the plate. It displaces the esoteric food pyramid, which might have been a gift from aliens visiting ancient Egypt.

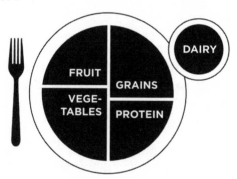

These new *Dietary Guidelines* pretty well mirror our recommendations at Weight Watchers, emphasizing nutrient-dense and filling foods. A PointsPlus value is derived from a combination of protein, fats, carbohydrates, and sugar. In addition, fruits and vegetables are exempt from the PointsPlus value formula. Whole grains, lean proteins, and legumes—all fall gloriously low on the PointsPlus scale.

But again, knowing what to eat is a far cry from actually eating the right foods day in and day out.

That's why I turn to certain additional insights that I have found helpful for more intuitively making good choices and sticking with a sustainable weight loss and maintenance plan.

# INSIGHT #1: YOU CAN'T BEAT THE FIRST LAW OF THERMODYNAMICS

The first and most important point about losing or maintaining weight is that the first law of thermodynamics always holds true. In other words:

An increase in internal energy of a system =
heat supplied to the system – work done on the system

"Why of course!" you're saying. "Why didn't someone tell me sooner?" The translation of this in our midsections can be thought of simply as:

Calories retained (in the fat layer) =
calories consumed (food) – calories burned (exercise)

Burn more calories than you eat, and you lose. Maintain equilibrium and you stay the same. Eat too much or exercise too little, and you gain. Let's take this equation apart.

The calories burned part is a little tricky. The calories our bodies burn each day can be thought of as the sum of:

**1.** The simple functioning of our body just to keep us alive (i.e., breathing, sleeping, circulating blood, etc.). This basic level of body activity is known as the resting metabolic rate.

**2.** The energy we use performing our daily tasks: running down to (or away from) the boss's office, doing errands, wandering around the house, etc. If you do manual labor or are on your feet all day, this can add up to a substantial burn. For most of us, lots of household activities can indeed burn calories, but maybe not always as much as we think.

**3.** Add 1 and 2 and you've got about 90 percent of your calorie burn for the day.

The "calories consumed" part is pretty straightforward. All food contains energy that is ultimately converted into blood sugars and used by the body. Different foods contain different amounts of energy, and this can be seen in caloric content on food labels. Pretty basic stuff.

Here is the first cold hard truth about losing weight: It is really difficult to lose weight purely through exercise. Unless you are doing a fairly massive amount of exercise, it's a lot easier to inadvertently eat 500 extra calories than it is to burn 500 calories. I can burn up several hundred calories in a brutal 50-minute Spinning class, but I'm a heaving mess by the time it's over. It goes without saying that before I became an active exerciser, I was not doing vigorous activity like this. More likely, I would be doing moderate pace walking for an hour, which would be good for a couple hundred calories at my weight. That works out to about half of a typical scone. In other words, it's 2 hours to burn off that scone. Perhaps it would be better not to eat either half of the scone in the first place?

To lose weight, most people, including me, need to reduce caloric intake. There is no way around it. I found that I was doing so much dumb, mindless eating that I was inhabiting what the military would call a target-rich environment. There were any number of lousy foods for me to give up. I had no choice but to start eating less and differently.

# INSIGHT #2: EAT BIG FOODS (WITH SMALL ENERGY DENSITY)

I am a volume eater. I grew up associating having lots of food with being satisfied. Eating four bites of anything and calling it a day does not fly with me. So I need to trick myself into thinking that I've had a lot of food. Fortunately, I am not alone.

Barbara Rolls, PhD, a professor of nutrition at Penn State University, and other researchers around the globe observed that most people are satisfied by the amount (i.e., volume) of food they eat rather than the calories in said food. This observation was a huge relief to me as it gave me a way to use sneaky tricks to evade the food devil. Their concept is built around the

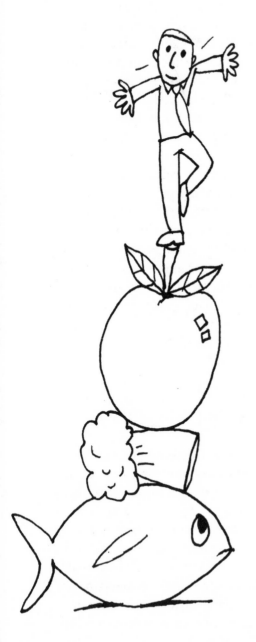

principle of energy density: Different foods have different numbers of calories (i.e., energy) per pound. If you were to eat 1 ounce of food that happened to contain 10 billion calories, you would surely turn into a supernova and explode. So don't do that.

Perhaps a more practical go-to example of energy density is this: grapes and raisins.

- ½ cup of raisins = 217 calories
- 4 (!) cups of grapes = 248 calories

Four cups of grapes would be pretty hard to eat in one sitting without feeling fairly foul afterward, but I could inhale half a cup of raisins and not even know it. What's going on here? Simple, one raisin has the same sugar as one grape, but a grape comes plumped out with a bunch of water. It creates a much greater sense of fullness.

Examples of foods I try to minimize or avoid because of excessive energy density include some obvious suspects such as butter and fat-heavy meats. I'm also careful around nuts, which offer great health benefits but are laden with calories (i.e., incredibly high energy density). To put it in perspective, 1 cup of pecans has 750 calories! I could eat a cup of pecans lickety-split and never know that I just ate the equivalent of nearly 1.5 Big Macs. So with nuts, let's keep the snack to a healthy handful (about 23 almonds, for 163 calories).

Or take a look at oranges versus orange juice. One orange has about 60 calories; an 8-ounce glass of orange juice has about 110 calories. It has never taken me more than 3.4 seconds to drink 8 ounces of orange juice, while an orange actually takes a few minutes to eat. Plus there's all that exercise in peeling the thing, then walking to the sink to wash my hands. Then somebody always asks if they can have a section or two . . .

This leads me to insight #3.

## INSIGHT #3: EAT FOOD THAT WILL SLOW YOUR JAWS DOWN

The juice versus fruit smack-down is an instructive one on a number of levels. When you eat the actual fruit, you are also consuming fiber, cellulose, and other noncaloric items that give a sense of fullness. The combination of these materials plus all of the water makes fruit a pretty attractive deal as far as energy density is concerned.

Plus all that tedious prep work involved at freeing a slice and conveying it to my mouth can take 10 minutes. Not so good for a tightly wound executive, but plenty good for a guy who has struggled with weight his whole adult life. If you take time to eat food, it gives your stomach a chance to start sending signals to the brain that it might be getting full. This would never happen with OJ; I could empty the carton, and my stomach would issue nary a peep.

# INSIGHT #4: EAT FOODS THAT STAY WITH YOU FOR A WHILE

In addition to energy density, nutritionists also talk about the concept of satiety. There is quite a bit of research out there that suggests that some foods are more naturally satisfying to our sense of hunger than others. For example, foods that are high in protein, like eggs, keep you fuller longer than foods that are high in carbohydrate, like a slice of toast. That's why most people can go longer without being hungry if they have eggs for breakfast instead of a piece of dry toast. By the way, fat provides the lowest satiety (and the most calories per gram) among the calorie-containing nutrients.

Through lots of diligent eating experiments to see if my satiety ratings track with what the research says, I have convinced myself that foods that include more protein and fiber also make me feel full longer.

# Putting It All Into Practice...

For me, the first trick was to replace my crummy food choices with much more intelligent ones. Let's start with my favorite example.

## HOW I REFORMED MY BREAKFAST

Going from a scary/unhealthy/artery-wrecking lifestyle to a healthier/happier/kinder lifestyle is not a simple process. I had to solve lots of food and exercise problems and make better choices. I approached this by hitting one habit cluster at a time. Each represented a dragon to slay and a kingdom to liberate. No, I haven't slain all of my dragons yet, but many of the most destructive ones have breathed their last high-calorie fire.

Breakfast is a good example. First off, breakfast is an incredibly important meal, so don't skip it. But eating breakfast used to mean I was getting into trouble not long after I got out of my pajamas. For years, I have been a regular Starbucks customer. I have an abused loyalty card to prove it. To its credit, Starbucks has worked hard to create some healthy food options for breakfast. I just didn't eat them. Instead, I worshipped at the altar of the coffee cake and the scone. I love pastry/muffins/breads of all sorts, and these guys make tasty ones. There's a reason they taste so great. As of today, their classic coffee cake clocks in at 440 calories (actually down from where it was a few years ago), while a blueberry scone has about 460 calories. Ouch!

With all of the best intentions, I moved on to a new breakfast food frontier in the form of a yogurt parfait sold by my local Pax Wholesome Foods chain. Hey, it's yogurt! It's got fruit! It must be a great deal! One 16-ounce serving dishes out about 400 calories. Despite the healthier appearances, this was only a slight improvement over Starbucks's carbohydrate bombs. I clearly had more work to do in finding a reliably good and satisfying breakfast.

So I started with some basic, solid principles and evolved my breakfasts over time. Here are my better breakfast release notes. (I'm back to my computer metaphors, so watch out):

- **Better breakfast 1.0:** Quaker flavored oatmeal, Dannon Fruit on the Bottom yogurt, and coffee with sugar and 2% milk. This wasn't a terrible version 1.0, but it clearly contained a bunch of bugs. For example, standard flavored oatmeal has lots of added sugar and flavors that may or may not be natural. I'm not puritanical about the whole organic food thing, but there were still too many calories in this version.

- **Better breakfast 2.0:** Quaker Weight Control oatmeal, Dannon Light & Fit yogurt. Better, particularly since this oatmeal has more protein. Still, not enough food to keep me full until lunch.

- **Better breakfast 3.0**: Quaker Weight Control oatmeal with banana and blueberries added. Also for this release is the introduction of Chobani 0% Greek yogurt with fruit. I have become a giant Greek yogurt convert: more protein than conventional yogurt and not too many calories in the 0% fat variety. Still, I was sensing that there was an opportunity to cut down even further on the added sugar.

- **Better breakfast 4.0:** McCann's unflavored instant oatmeal plus fruit. Fage Total 0% plain yogurt plus grapes. This breakfast gives me enough food to be thoroughly satisfied without blowing my food allowance for the rest of the day.

Breakfast 4.0 is perfect for me. It's a ton of food without any useless added sugar. I am endlessly amused that I can take a little packet of oatmeal and turn it into a giant bowl of breakfast food through the miracle of fruit bulking. The result? I am almost never hungry until lunch.

# FIXING MY LUNCH

Somewhere in the mid-2000s, I slipped into a really bad habit that many of us Weight Watchers vets fall into: thinking I know more than I actually do. Rather than looking up what was in foods, I would eyeball menu items and tell myself that they weren't such bad choices. One day I grew suspicious of my assumptions and downloaded the nutritional data from a local place I frequented (Yes, I really am that much of a geek.)

What I found was pretty scary. Let's take the innocent-sounding California Wrap. Could it really be that bad? Aren't all Californians thin, blond, and tan? Well, in this case, the apparently virtuous combination of "grilled chicken, lettuce, tomatoes, fresh avocado, and roasted peppers with Thousand Island dressing in a whole wheat wrap" works out to 700 calories. I compounded the mistake by ordering blueberry yogurt parfait made with "plump blueberries and toasted granola blended with low-fat blueberry yogurt," which totaled 410 calories. It made for a whopping 29 PointsPlus values out of my total of 41 per day. This was bad math, and it proved my eye for nutrition was even worse.

One decision I made was to fully embrace salad as a lunch mainstay. As someone who grew up with bread-overload lunches, I found this a bit of a change. I ultimately came to the conclusion that I did not want to spend my daily target on bread or wraps. I declared the salad to be a sandwich without bread. Here is what I like about salad: It looks like a lot of food, and it takes a while to eat. I like the fact that I don't have to skimp on goodies such as meats and friendly vegetables, and I even get a little cheese.

Here is a typical salad I'll eat at lunch on a workday:

- Turkey
- Spinach
- A little bit of shredded Cheddar cheese
- Vegetables like chickpeas, mushrooms, and sweet potatoes
- Fat-free dressing

When you see it assembled, it may not be the prettiest thing in the world, with too many earth tones. But it's tasty, filling, and leaves me in good shape for the rest of the day. Again, this is the same theory: lots of protein and volume resulting in a happy stomach—and, by the way, I also think it tastes great. Contrast this to my wrap plus yogurt parfait, and I'm consuming one-third the calories but getting all of the fullness and satisfaction. Plus seeing a ton of food is beyond sexy in my simple mind.

## MAKING MY DINNER DECENT

When it comes to dinner, I have it easy. My wife is a wonderful cook, and she can translate dietary disasters into healthy recipes, often using her "secret": that most dishes can be made with a fraction of the oil called for in the recipe, with no loss of taste. I am routinely treated to tasty low-fat meals that fall well within my intake range. Thanks, sweetie.

So what are these magical meals? I eat lots of seafood with a smattering of chicken dishes and the occasional pork loin. They come equipped with large sides of vegetables. I still have pasta, but it is now delivered in normal portion sizes and without the Alfredo sauce of old.

So what happens when she's not looking out for me? The easiest meal for a guy to prepare is something on the grill. Grilled meats and vegetables enjoy the benefit of little to no oil, and they are almost purely unprocessed foods (i.e., no hidden calories). You simply cannot go wrong with a skewer of meat or a grilled piece of chicken or fish (as long as it's not marinated in heavy oils or sauces). Match it up with some basic vegetable sides, and you are in great shape.

Overall, I have been able to fine-tune my meals such that I can pretty easily stay within my bounds, and I rarely have food blowups these days. Meals are no longer the places that get me in trouble.

# SNACKING AND GRAZING: BEING AWARE OF TRIGGER FOODS

We all have a set of foods that make us weak in the knees, are full of calories, taste amazing, and are actively working toward our nutritional demise. We call them trigger foods. Here's how the WeightWatchers.com Web site defines them:

> A trigger food is a specific food that sets off a course of overeating where control is lost and excessive amounts are consumed. The most common trigger foods are sugar/fat combinations (ice cream, cookies) and fat/salt combinations (nuts, potato chips). Food triggers are fairly uncommon and should not be confused with favorite foods (foods that are highly preferred), comfort foods (foods that are linked to a sense of home and contentment),

or food cravings (desire for a food that has not been consumed in a long time). With a true food trigger, it is the food, not an emotion or a situation, that triggers the out-of-control eating. For example, open the bag of potato chips and it will be gone, regardless of your mood, the time of day, or the place.

We all have our own trigger foods. What sends one person into a freakish eating frenzy might garner nothing more than a "meh" from someone else. I have spent some time thinking about my triggers, and here are the ones I'll pull almost every time:

- **Hummus:** Deadly stuff for me, even though it is a perfectly honorable food. Set me up with a tub of this and a box of Reduced Fat Triscuits and watch the crumbs fly. I can easily run through 12 to 15 Triscuits and a half tub of Sabra. I can pack away a third of my day's calorie allowance in about 5 minutes of mindless munching.

- **Pretzels:** I started eating pretzels instead of chips because they seemed the healthier option (not fried). When I go this way, I often use honey mustard as a dipping agent. Again, my logic here is that it is a healthier way to go. Typical outing? Sixteen Rold Gold Honey Wheat Braided Twists and 4 tablespoons Honeycup Uniquely Sharp Mustard. Not as bad as the hummus, but it still qualifies for "meal" status and isn't just a snack.

- **Reduced-calorie ice cream treats:** This is a classic example of completely abusing a product designed to help you. I almost never have just one Weight Watchers ice cream treat; I usually opt to go double fisted. Yes, portion control is a great way to manage food intake, but you've got to stop with the portion you're supposed to have.

- **Nuts:** It is disturbing how much I like nuts. All nuts of all types, which is unfortunate given their calorie density. The defined portion (in other words, the amount that a reasonable person would eat in one sitting) is ½ cup of almonds, or 30 nuts. The issue, as always, is portion control. For me, an open bag of nuts is soon an empty bag of nuts.

What I find striking about my list is that most people would say that these foods are good components for healthy (or at least not fully unhinged) snacking. Yet it's always a matter of degree: In my unsteady hands they do great damage.

So how can I keep my finger off the trigger foods? For the most part, I try to avoid them. I know I'm a compulsive eater, so when I'm in the company of these foods, I'm not quite myself. I can limit the damage by preportioning the foods: Never, ever eat directly from the container! And a reduced-calorie ice-cream treat is on the right track: It's a single serving, so there's less temptation, but I really should have it with my dinner, not idly sitting on the couch watching TV. However, for the most part, I need to say no to some of these foods—not because they are bad foods, but because my brain has a bad interaction with them.

I had to find a whole new crew of snack-food friends to keep me out of trouble. If trigger foods are my sworn enemies, which foods can be my new upstanding friends? Here are some basic criteria:

**1. They should take a while to eat.** Food works best if it can meet a basic time criteria and create the sensation that you've had meaningful eating experience. If it can be eaten in three bites, it is not a true snacking friend. Tiresome acquaintance at best.

**2. They should look larger than life.** That is, the food should occupy a significant amount of space and create the illusion that it is a boatload of food. Of course, it should be an optical illusion of sorts, as it should also have a limited number of calories. In Weight Watchers lingo, these are referred to as Filling Foods.

**3. They should taste good and stay in my belly for a long time.** If I can savor it, and it produces the holy state of satiety—nothing more for me, thanks, I'm full—then we're really getting somewhere.

So let me introduce you to these new pals, who keep me out of trouble when my hands are idle and my stomach is rumbling.

## My New Snack Friends

- **Apples:** Particularly Fuji apples. I also appreciate that one apple can be sliced into eighths, which equals two bites each. That's 16 bites of food and only 100 calories—an excellent deal.

- **Fat-free Greek yogurt:** Not awesome by itself, but it plays very nicely with others. It also contains lots of protein with relatively few calories, so it takes time to digest. A 6-ounce container of Fage Total 0% Greek yogurt contains 18 grams of protein (!) but only 100 calories. This is my definition of an amazing deal. I have been known to organize playdates between Greek yogurt and an apple.

- **Grapes:** I have a friend who calls grapes "nature's candy," and he's right on the money. I love the taste, and they take a long time to eat. Which is good. Grapes also go nicely with the aforementioned slightly boring Greek yogurt.

- **94% fat-free microwave popcorn:** This is another snack food that takes a lot of time to consume yet has very few tag-along calories to go with the experience. And no, melted butter is not on the invite list, regardless of whether you add it yourself or it's already in the bag.

- **Salsa 'n' vegetables:** Don't dis the crudités. They may not be manly, but they are a more than suitable substitution for chips and crackers. I love dipping, so throw some salsa into the mix, and I'm a happy camper. Mix the veggies up beyond the usual boring celery and carrot sticks. Mushrooms, broccoli, cauliflower, asparagus, sweet peppers, and jicama keep my stomach and mouth occupied and help me rack up extra vegetables in my diet.

- **Bean dip:** I love hummus, and I was sorry to unfriend it. But bean dip has a scary-good calorie value, because most brands are processed without oil.

## SPECIAL TOPIC #1: In praise of the least-appreciated snack on Earth, jerky

Dial the clock back to 1983, when *Trading Places* appeared on movie screens across the United States. My favorite scene (if I am forced to choose) is the one in which Billy Ray Valentine (Eddie Murphy), Louis Winthorpe III (Dan Aykroyd), Ophelia (Jamie Lee Curtis—looking great), and Coleman (Denholm Elliott) are attempting to recover the orange juice crop report from the dastardly Clarence Beeks (the amazing Paul Gleason).

> **BILLY RAY, DISGUISED AS NAGA EBOKO IN AFRICAN GARB, SAYS HELLO TO COLEMAN, DISGUISED AS A PRIEST:** "Beef jerky?"
>
> **COLEMAN/PRIEST:** "No, son, it gives me wind something terrible."

These lines were etched in my mind for the next quarter of a century. How could they make such a thing up, even in a movie? It must be true. For 25 years, I couldn't look at jerky without grimacing.

Two years ago, I gave myself a long hard look in the mirror. I asked the wrenching question that I had been avoiding for so many years: Was I willing to recognize cheap, tawdry stereotypes foisted on innocent foods, by Hollywood no less? With tears streaming down my cheeks, I accepted the truth: I had given jerky a bum rap, and dammit, it deserved better. It was time to give it an open-minded try. I bought some Trader Joe's buffalo and turkey jerky, and chewed. And chewed. And chewed. Conclusion: Both tasted fantastic, and I was no windier than usual. Another stereotype crushed!

One might reasonably ask, who cares? I do. Here is why beef jerky matters: few calories, many grams of protein. This translates into snacking and satiety glory. One serving of jerky typically has 70 calories and 14 grams of protein in a 1.1-ounce serving. In addition, jerky takes a while to eat because it is hard and chewy. It's almost the perfect snack, if you're okay eating dried animals. And even though it contains a lot of sodium, I can enjoy it without going overboard on the salt-o-meter.

## SPECIAL TOPIC #2: Do I commit fruit abuse?

I was invited on FoxBusiness television in the fall of 2011 to talk about obesity and health care. While I was getting miked up, one of the guys on the Fox crew gave me the secret guy-in-Weight-Watchers handshake. We are a brave group of pioneers, and our numbers are rapidly increasing. This particular guy shared with me that his one concern about the bro-gram was that fruit had zero PointsPlus values—meaning that in theory you could eat as much of it as you want. He was nervous about going overboard and perhaps had done a little of that.

I feel your pain, brother!

I tried to assuage his fears of a banana binge. I told him that it's actually pretty hard to go crazy on fruit. (If anybody could have done so, it would have been me.) While fruit does have natural sugars, it is also packed with fiber and water, so it's naturally filling. Plus, if you really did go all fruit bat and eat the whole bunch of bananas, the repercussions downstream would be dramatic and unpleasant. (Biointestinal feedback, right?) Finally, I told him that while fruit had a zero PointsPlus value, as do most vegetables, we warn people not to treat it as a mindless eating/binge food. Don't suspend reality. It is in fact hard to lose weight while eating 73 apples a day.

I love fruit—almost to an unnatural degree—so if bingeing starts with love, I am at risk. However, I can stomach only about five servings of fruit on a typical day. Here is the tally:

- **Grapes:** 1½ cups = 90 calories (22 g carbs, 2 g fiber, 1 g protein, 0 g fat). Like most fruit, the grape is mostly water and pulp.

- **Banana:** 1 large = 121 calories (32 g carbs, 3.5 g fiber, 1.5 g protein, 0 g fat). Bananas are a bit of a watch-out food for me because they go down a little too fast; I usually only eat them sliced up in my oatmeal.

- **Blueberries:** ½ cup = 41 calories (10 g carbs, 2 g fiber, 1 g protein, 0 g fat). These guys are a pretty great deal. Raspberries are an even better deal (32 calories for the same ½ cup).

- **Apple:** 1 medium = 95 calories (25 g carbs, 4.4 g fiber, 0.5 g protein, 0 g fat). They take a while to eat, and they're pretty filling.

- **MY FRUIT FILL FOR THE DAY:** 347 calories (89 g carbs, 12 g fiber, 4 g protein, 0 g fat).

Looking at the math makes me feel even better about my fruit fancy. It's an awful lot of food, and it's a big reason why I don't spend my days battling hunger pangs.

Moral of the story for me? Just because fruit has zero PointsPlus values doesn't mean throwing mindfulness out the window. Tracking can be good, even when you find out you're adding up a bunch of zeros.

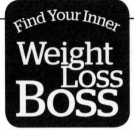

# When it comes to food, keep it simple—and keep it satisfying

## Remember the law of thermodynamics.

Weight loss comes down to a simple equation: calories in (food) versus calories out (exercise and activity). It would have been impossible for me to lose the weight I did with exercise alone. In fact, I believe I lost most of my weight by reducing my caloric input, not by increasing my caloric output.

## Don't make it too complicated.

Stick to the basic tenets of the Dietary Guidelines for Americans' plate: Fill half the plate with fruits and vegetables, and the rest with lean proteins and whole grains. Wash it down with low-fat milk, and you're good.

## Do your research.

Don't assume that a food is your friend just because it sounds healthy. Look up its caloric and nutritional values first.

## Choose big foods.

And slow foods. And filling foods. Some people like to get a lot of food for their $5. I like to get a lot of food for my 200 calories. To do that, focus on bulk (salads), satiety (oatmeal with fruit), and foods you just can't eat too much of. (Ever have more than one apple? No!)

## Don't pull your triggers.

Identify the foods that trigger big feeds, then run in the opposite direction. Snack on foods that you're less likely to eat in mass quantities (celery sticks, not pretzel rods). Most important, find alternatives to your trigger foods. It's much easier to replace a not-so-helpful food with a good one than it is to simply stop eating the not-so-helpful food.

## Find staple meals that are habit-forming.

I love my standard breakfast—the aforementioned oatmeal with fruit. I also love that I don't have to think about what to have for breakfast. It's automatic. In a world where there are at least five flavors of Coke, you need to limit the field. Sample widely, choose well, lock it in, and your world just became a whole lot simpler. Not having to make choices can mean not having to make not-so-good choices.

## Weight Watchers Profile

## "Live like you were dying."

A Tim McGraw song title proves frighteningly true—and terrifically motivating

**Erin Meyer, 28,** *Olathe, KS*

**HEIGHT:** 6 feet 1 inch
**WEIGHT BEFORE:** 420
**WEIGHT AFTER:** 210
Reached her goal in 5 years

### MY STRUGGLE

I was always the overweight kid growing up. In fifth or sixth grade, when my weight gain really accelerated, I was already 5 foot 10 and over 200 pounds. I was a solid kid—and I knew nothing about healthy eating. I thought I was making a good choice by eating a salad, but I'd smother it in full-fat dressing and buttered veggies. I tried to control my weight with crash diets, which only led to more weight gain.

### MY WAKE-UP CALL

On Memorial Day in 2006, when I weighed my most, I was in a car accident that snapped my right leg in half at the knee. When my doctor looked at me and said, "You physically cannot walk again without losing weight.

Your body just won't sustain it, and your leg can't heal otherwise." I knew I had to change my life. I couldn't imagine being handicapped forever. It just wasn't an option. I thought, How bad do I really want to live life? And what kind of life do I really want to live?

### MY FOOD

Instead of my normal crash-diet approach, I took a long time to lose the weight and learned to alter my favorite foods along the way. For example, when I make baked ziti, I use Ronzoni Smart Taste pasta and lower-calorie tomato sauce, then add sautéed onions, zucchini, tomatoes, and peppers. As for maintaining my weight, I've learned to set realistic expectations, so I don't break down and binge. When I went to a conference in New Orleans for 9 days, I decided, "I'm going to work out in the morning. I'm going to do my best at breakfast and lunch. Dinner doesn't matter." If I allow myself to indulge, I always make up for it elsewhere.

## MY FITNESS

After being told that I'd never walk again, running a 5-K became one of my goals. I don't have any cartilage in my right knee, and I have arthritis after the accident. I've already been told that I'll need a total replacement around age 35 and that I'm not allowed to run after I hit 30. So for me, it's become a question of "Well, what are things I was told I'd never be able to do that I can accomplish now?" So I trained, and I did my first 5-K. Then I was able to do a 10-K. Now I'm training for a half-marathon.

For me, goal setting is huge. If you take the time to write down what you want to change, how it will benefit you, and how you're going to achieve it, you'll have more motivation to stick with it. There's a great quote by Benjamin Mays, the great educator and mentor to Martin Luther King Jr.: "The tragedy of life does not lie in not reaching your goal. The tragedy in life is having no goal to reach." If you don't ever bother setting goals, you have nothing to work for.

## MY PAYOFF

I feel like I'm living for the first time. I never could have imagined that I'd be as happy as I am now. Or that I'd have my master's in education and would be teaching full-time. Or that I'd be running 10-Ks, training for a half-marathon, and would actually be able to start dating. I feel like Tim McGraw's song "Live Like You Were Dying." I nearly did, but Weight Watchers gave me the gift of health.

# {CHAPTER 5}

# Rely on Habits, Not Willpower–

## The Secret to Success

 **HAD THE NUTRITIONAL IQ OF A BLOCK OF WOOD** when I started with Weight Watchers. Still, I found it pretty easy to learn the basics about good foods and not-so-good ones. If obesity was simply a function of nutritional knowledge, the obesity epidemic would have vanished at the end of Chapter 4.

If only it were that easy.

Once again, the hard part in losing weight and keeping it off isn't knowing what to do. The hard part is making it happen in your life.

Let's start with the fundamentals. We live in an environment that conspires against us. We are surrounded by mountains of food and oceans of drinks, and the large corporations that produce them are killing themselves to sell you more, more, MORE. They come up with catchy slogans, arresting package designs, irresistible aromas, palate explosions, and crave-worthy concoctions, and then they hire sexy actresses and hunky athletes to wave it all at you and beckon you to eat, eat, EAT. We are constantly tempted and tested with 24/7 access to as much cheap food as we could ever hope to consume. This plague of plenty comes at a time when our personal energy expenditures are at an all-time low. Most of us no longer do manual labor, so we're sitting ducks for weight gain.

But it's not just too much food and too little movement. Many of us, me included, eat for reasons that have nothing to do with being hungry. We eat to celebrate, and we eat because there's nothing to celebrate. We eat because we're happy and because we're unhappy. We shovel it down during the excitement of the *American Idol* finale or during the boredom of reruns. You can argue that we even use food to self-medicate—a pint of ice cream to salve the pain of a breakup or the stress of a tough job.

There is a lot of very interesting research, discussed later in the book, about how our brain lights up like a Christmas tree when we see what looks like tasty food. We are constantly having to battle a lot of neurologic impulses in our efforts to resist temptation or to leave some food on our plates.

Ultimately, most of our food and activity behaviors are habits, many of which we developed early in our lives. Some of our habits are healthy (exercise before breakfast!) and some of them are not so healthy (doughnuts with coffee!).

In the context of this, I'm often irritated when I hear people say that managing weight is a function of discipline and willpower. It's as though we can hope to deal with our weight issues only if we happen to have superhero character traits. This line of reasoning suggests that a dietary lapse or failed weight loss attempt is a function of a personal flaw or weakness. That couldn't be further from the truth, and frankly it hurts people's chance of success. None of us is perfect 100 percent of the time—certainly not the CEO of Weight Watchers. But if we can up our success rate from 60 to 85 percent, point by point, we can achieve great things in life. No sense in beating yourself up over the failures that you're bound to have.

The key for me in addressing my weight issue was staying focused on the notion of trying to form new healthier habits. Here are my biggest personal insights into the entire weight discussion.

**1.** The only way to sustainably lose weight is to adopt a healthier lifestyle.

**2.** A healthy lifestyle is simply a bunch of healthy habits.

**3.** Healthy habits are hard to acquire, but we can do it if we think about them the right way.

So your process is much less about memorizing a list of foods or becoming an expert on high-fructose corn syrup, and more about cultivating healthy habits. We need to establish an environment that helps us foster those habits. We need to recognize that the key to forming habits is repetition. And finally, we need to cut ourselves a little slack when our habit-forming virtues take a turn toward vice.

# How to Form a Good Habit—for Good

So what exactly is a habit? I found the following definition in *Psychology Today*, and it seems as good as any.

> Habit formation is the process by which new behaviors become automatic. If you instinctively reach for a cigarette the moment you wake up in the morning, you have a habit. By the same token, if you lace up your running shoes and hit the streets as soon as you get home, you've acquired a habit. Old habits are hard to break, and new habits are hard to form. That's because the behavioral patterns we repeat most often are literally etched in our neural pathways. The good news is that through repetition, it's possible to form new habits.

By its very definition, a habit is something you really don't think much about. It's pretty automatic. A good habit doesn't require willpower or discipline, you just do it. With a bad habit, you probably don't think about what you are doing until you are doing it or until you suffer the repercussions. (Like when that nurse kept on moving the weights left on the scale, during my crucial doctor visit. Haunting.) If you're stuck on autopilot, you never have a chance to institute willpower or discipline, for better or worse.

Your simple goal is this: (1) establish healthy habits, and (2) eliminate unhealthy habits. It takes work—that's the bad news. The good news is that it's absolutely doable if you set yourself up for success. And that means managing expectations around what success looks like.

Forging new habits takes time and repetition. You can't install one like you would a new dishwasher. I haven't been able to fully commit to a new habit in less than 2 months, and some of my habits have taken 6 to 12 months to really internalize.

Because I know that habit formation is a process rather than an instant pudding, I recognize that any new habit will likely take a few attempts, including a few failures. When I fail, I try again and don't bother beating myself up repeatedly.

Also, we think we've established a new habit or licked an old one, but we're always at risk for backsliding. When it happens, we have choices: (1) fall into a heap of despair and disgust, or (2) pick ourselves up and reapply ourselves. No, it's not easy to recover from recidivism, but when I was flagellating myself, I wished someone had given me this pep talk.

How does one establish a new habit? What has to be in place for the effort to succeed? How do we create an environment that tilts us to success? What tools can we employ to improve our odds of success?

First off, your head has to be in the game. I want to refer you again to the research that Weight Watchers did a decade ago on people who had successful weight loss attempts, regardless of whether they were following our program or someone else's. The winners almost universally shared the following qualities:

**1.** They had a sense of urgency. Losing the weight really mattered to them, and it was a top 5 priority.

**2.** They had a sense of belief that if they simply stuck with whatever program they were following, they would ultimately succeed.

Think of the opposite of these two conditions. Hypothetically, if I have just gotten divorced, lost my job, seen one of my kids get hooked on crystal meth, and let my parents move into my house, losing weight might not be the number-one issue at this moment. I wouldn't be able to lose weight because I would have too many other priorities that would crush it like a bug on a windshield. By the same token, if my mind-set at the start is "I will probably fail like I have so many times before, but I guess I should try again," then I will probably fail because I've already preordained the outcome.

As I've written, I had two triggers that made losing weight a priority. One was getting grief from my doctor, and the second was taking a job at Weight Watchers. You don't need those triggers to have a sense of urgency. But you will have to come to this realization: Losing weight matters enough that you'll gut it out when you might otherwise quit.

In terms of my own confidence, I just trusted that Weight Watchers could work for me because it had for so many others. You may be thinking, Of course he'd say that. He's the CEO! But I'm not just shilling for my company, and I have the results to prove it. The whole approach of getting weigh-ins, counting Points, etc., made intuitive sense to me, and when I saw other people in the Weight Watchers meeting scoring successes, I wanted a piece of the action. I'm silly competitive. There was no way I was going to watch someone else succeed and not get the same for myself.

# THE FORMULA FOR BEHAVIOR CHANGE

There is a lot of research under way in the field of behavior modification (i.e., the science of habits), and I've been fortunate to meet many of the scientists. Among them: a researcher out of Stanford named B. J. Fogg, PhD, a superinteresting guy who spends his time thinking about how we change habits. He came up with a model, the Fogg Behavior Model, that I think really explains the dynamic.

Okay, it's a little geeky, but I like geeky things. Here are the key elements of this diagram.

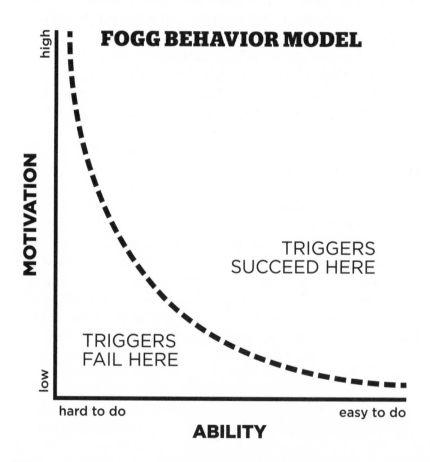

**1. Motivation:** Generically, a motivator can be pleasure, pain, hope, fear, social acceptance, or social rejection.

**2. Ability:** To make a change, you have to be able to do it. According to B.J., the simpler the task you set for yourself, the more likely your ability will kick in.

**3. Trigger:** A trigger can be external (i.e., an alarm clock or a personal trainer or a Weight Watchers leader) or internal (i.e., a routine we have established). Triggers are basically the electric shocks that stimulate our action.

I think of the three factors coming together as a chemical reaction, in which you need all three to make something happen. A chemical reaction requires two reagents and generally a catalyst (like heat) to make your beaker blow up. Behavior change is similar.

Here's how I think of B.J.'s framework in relation to my own change process.

**1. Motivators:** How do I create goals, desirable outcomes, incentives, and other tricks to help me stay focused in my efforts?

**2. Ability:** What steps can I take to make this whole process easier to stick with? For example, how can I change my environment?

**3. Triggers:** What makes me lose it around food? I'm a fool for an open bag, box, or carton. I lust after ice cream, nuts, and dips. I know, so I don't go there. Usually.

Let's put it all together. If there is a habit I'm trying to shed, I first need to be motivated to lose the bad habit. I will need an incentive or reward to make the effort worthwhile. If it is, I then need a simple way or mechanism to shed the habit so that it is not the equivalent of climbing Mount Everest. The habit should be a small enough and/or simple enough change so that I can actually make it happen. Finally, I need some kind of trigger to spur me into action.

So where am I today in the habit change continuum? I am far from complete, but I'm also much better off from where I started in 2000. As I noted above, I've now got breakfast down to a routine, and lunch and dinner usually proceed without any big missteps. I also exercise regularly, which I'll discuss in Chapter 6.

There are other good habits I've developed over the past 10 years that I am probably not even aware of. That's when you know you've locked in positive change: You don't even realize you're doing it. If, every day, I had to make the decision to exercise or to have a decent breakfast, I would inevitably revert back to my former heavier self.

So do I have it all figured out? Absolutely not. To this day, I still have my running inventory of not-so-great habits that I would really like to get rid of.

# BAD HABITS I'D LIKE TO LOSE

## BAD HABIT #1: Sneaking—Man as Child

As a Lifetime Member of Weight Watchers, I like to think of myself as the model of righteous living. Except when I am secretly not.

A few weeks ago, my wife and I were winding down after a typically long and busy day. She announced that she was going upstairs, and I told her I'd be up in just a little bit. After I heard her go up, I headed over to the freezer in something of a frenzy. There was ice cream in them there hills! I quick-drew a spoon as if it were a concealed weapon and dug deep into the vat of low-fat Edy's. The spoon flashed from carton to mouth. And that's when my wife walked into the kitchen. Caught!

She had a good laugh at me, noting that I looked like a 7-year-old boy with a hand in the cookie jar. She asked why I wouldn't just put the ice cream in a bowl and eat it like a normal person. Good question, and kind of a humiliating one at that.

Why do I sneak food? Had I merely had some ice cream in broad daylight, no one would have thought anything of it. You can certainly do this (in moderation) under the Weight Watchers program. What is it about sneaking that almost makes the food taste better? Why do I sneak now when I know that I will suffer (guilt, weight gain) later?

As I've already confessed, I've been a sneaker since childhood. When I was growing up, my bedroom was next door to the basement, where we kept our food-storage freezer containing my mother's large inventory of frozen bread, plus various staples. As a little boy, I used to sneak frozen bread (as I write this, it's hard for me to believe that I'm not making it up). Never mind that I could have gone upstairs and had a thawed piece of bread. The frozen, stolen slice just tasted better to me.

My mother used to bake tin after tin of Christmas cookies in early December, then stick them in the freezer—next to the frosty bread—until the holidays. Yes! It was like storing the gold bullion next to Butch and Sundance's lair. I would carry out stealth cookie removal, which involved intricate rearrangement of the cookies within the tins so that the loss was imperceptible. I discovered years later that she knew all along I was nabbing cookies. She just didn't say anything since the shrinkage was at manageable levels.

I did the same with ice cream, painstakingly scraping the top 3 millimeters off the surface of the container. Busted again. I ultimately outgrew the freezer raids, but I never outgrew the sneak mentality.

Secretive eating remains one of my weaknesses. Why? I think it's the thrill of forbidden fruit with a dash of furtive embarrassment. There is a freedom to self-indulgence, especially if you don't have to worry about recrimination or shaming. But can we ever actually fool ourselves? Nope.

Here are a few strategies I've developed for thwarting this kind of hidden habit.

## Steps to Stop Sneaking

**1.** Hang out your dirty laundry in a safe environment where others will relate and be supportive. (Starting a blog, notifying your Facebook friends, or attending a Weight Watchers meeting are good places to start.) In 1961, our founder Jean Nidetch sought similar support when she held the first ever Weight Watchers meeting in her apartment in Queens, New York. The mutual support and empathy that was enjoyed that night is the whole reason Weight Watchers exists today.

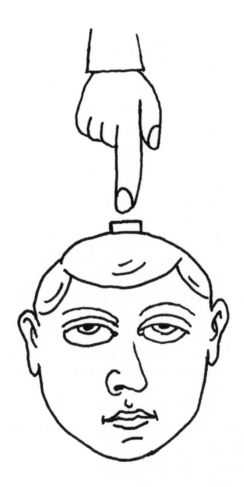

**2.** Find ways to focus less on what others think and more on what works for you. I need healthy behaviors for myself, not for the approval of others.

**3.** Understand that going undercover with minor indulgences encourages them to blossom into monstrous food disasters. Shame is its own weird kind of motivation.

**4.** Become more aware of the situations in which you're tempted to sneak food, and find detours—or major highways—around them.

**5.** Plan indulgences into your routine so they don't knock you off your path of progress. Then it's a pothole, not a crevasse.

# BAD HABIT #2: Grazing–Man as Cow

If I were ever stuck in a field for an extended period of time, I think I'd eventually start grazing on grass. I may actually have three additional stomachs, in the bovine way. I totally get cows, and I understand why they graze. I attribute their contented mien to the fact that they get to eat all the time.

Or maybe they're just bored? I know how that goes because I am a boredom eater. Give me a jam-packed day and I stick to my three square meals. It's almost as if I have good sense. But on a slow Saturday around the house, I'm always prowling around the kitchen. It's even worse if I'm slightly sleep deprived. I'm not hungry, yet I am deriving curious pleasure from masticating small handfuls of food.

To be clear, I should make the distinction between grazing and snacking. I define a snack as a small meal, which is often planned and deliberate. Grazing is merely the act of continuing to eat a little bit at a time in a continuous loop.

Grazing has not been an easy habit for me to kick. The Weight Watchers PointsPlus system has given me a simple guide to replacing bad foods with better ones, disastrous meals with healthy and satisfying ones. I've been able to incorporate those strategies quite easily into my day, and I stick with them. The meals come at the same intervals, and they're just good for me, not bad. But beating grazing has been hard because it requires not just replacing a food, but not eating at all when I want to. What to do? As I see it, I have a few choices.

## Steps to Stop Grazing

**1.** Find some other activity to replace it. We tell members this all the time. "When you are feeling bored, why not _____?" My problem is that I cannot for the life of me figure out what _____ is. Turn somersaults? Perfect my French accent? Calculate long-form algebra? Take up meditation, possibly combined with Yogic flying?

**2.** Replace the questionable grazing provisions (e.g., nuts) with smarter choices (e.g., carrot sticks, fruit).

**3.** Track Points values—or calories or handfuls—more actively. Do this particularly after dinner and on weekends. As they say, what gets measured gets done. And those handfuls of junk I eat when bored should count, too. Maybe double.

**4.** Plan snacks instead of grazing. The more I make conscious food choices, the better off I generally am. If I know that I'm having a snack, then it can remind me not to randomly grab food from the kitchen.

Mindless eating is the bane of many of our efforts to live more healthfully. Grazing is the most obvious example of mindless eating, but others exist as well. (More on this later.)

### BAD HABIT #3: The Clean Plate Club

Many of us remember our mothers saying, "If you don't finish your dinner, a thousand small children in Africa will starve." Or perhaps you were one of those kids who got the "You can have dessert only if I can wipe a white glove across your plate" treatment.

The first point to keep in mind is that the plates we were cleaning back then were typically 9 inches in diameter versus

12 inches today. If this doesn't sound like a big deal, consider that a 9-inch plate has a surface area of 63.5 square inches versus 113 square inches for a 12-inch plate. Therefore, emptying that plate back in the '60s and '70s involved half the load it does today.

But now, as adults, we clean it voluntarily. And when I clean a plate, it is squeaky clean. Who needs a dishwasher?

There are three solutions here.

## Steps to Stop Cleaning Your Plate

**1.** Shop a yard sale for some '70s-era dishware, and while you're at it, shrink the glasses, too. We're conditioned to empty the plate and drain the tankard, and if they're too big, we'll be too big as well.

**2.** Serve your portion in the kitchen. The old idea of serving up loaded platters family style is a simple invitation to eat every last scrap. And that's an invitation we're likely to accept.

**3.** Remind yourself to leave a third to a fourth of your food on the plate at the end of the meal. I'm better at this in restaurants than I am at home, and when I succeed, I then give myself a sweet gold star and a big self-administered pat on the back.

# ESTABLISHING NEW HABITS VS. LOSING BAD ONES

As I work on changing bad behaviors, I've generally found it easier to establish a new habit or replace a bad habit with a better habit. Where I have struggled mightily is eliminating a habit and not replacing it with something better.

In truth, one way to think about habit change is to consider a key strategy for each type of desired change.

**Establishing a new habit:** Create a routine that can make the habit second nature. Making breakfast has become so automatic for me that I even lay out the food in almost exactly the same order, every morning. Repeat the same routine until you start doing it out of muscle memory.

**Getting rid of a bad habit:** Okay, it's hard to do. What has worked best for me has been to create mini-interventions. One example of this: Put calorie labels on trigger foods. The key is to create a heightened awareness so you can break out of a mindless state of action.

I'm not there yet, but it's at least nice to know that there are definitive steps I can take to keep whittling away. This healthy life game is for marathoners, not sprinters.

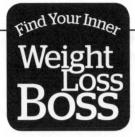

## Willpower is overrated. Instead, follow these keys to getting your life stuck on automatic.

## Focus your efforts on establishing healthy habits.

The beautiful aspect of a habit is that, by definition, it is something we do automatically. When we forge healthy habits, like having a good breakfast or taking a walk each day, we're more likely to stay on track because they are effortless. We are on autopilot. Establishing healthy habits isn't easy to do, but it is crucial. A couple tricks: (1) Make sure you have an incentive to do it, and (2) create a routine around it that makes it easier to work into your life.

## Pick your targets.

I have a list of bad habits in order of priority that I'd like to beat. Beating a bad habit is hard to do because it's so routine. I try to create some sort of intervention that makes me aware of the bad habit before I commit it. In other words, I turn off the autopilot by hitting the right switch. I also advise limiting the number of habits you try to tackle at any given time. Focus your efforts on two or three of them, and make them a priority.

## Backsliding happens.

As I mentioned, I'm not Superman. Or if I am, I keep on flying into the same buildings. Listen, we all fall off the wagon. Acknowledge it. Plan for it. And then climb back aboard—as if your life depended on it.

# Weight Watchers Profile

## "I've become a master at substitutions."

The most important one: swapping bad habits for good

**Carri Reiss, 30,** *Boston, MA*

**HEIGHT:** 5 feet 5 inches
**WEIGHT BEFORE:** 253
**WEIGHT AFTER:** 133
Reached her goal in 21 months

### MY STRUGGLE

I first became overweight around second or third grade, and at puberty I really blew up. I continued to gain weight through high school, college, and into adulthood. I joined Weight Watchers in high school for a week or two because my mom made me. Obviously, it didn't stick. I looked into prepackaged plans, but none seemed like they were for me. So I kept eating my favorite unhealthy foods. I'd order nachos covered with cheese, sour cream, and guacamole, then later that night would still eat a fairly large dinner.

### MY WAKE-UP CALL

In 2008, I had just moved to Boston, which is a walking city. It seemed like I was always the slowest person. My feet were hurting!

Around this time, I started having acid reflux and heartburn. I realized I needed a change—I couldn't keep living the way I always had. I asked my mom if she would like to join Weight Watchers with me. The next day, we both joined.

### MY FOOD

I've always enjoyed cooking, but my approach has changed a lot. I've become a master at substitutions. I replace part of the butter in recipes with fat-free chicken broth. When baking, I use applesauce instead of oil and eggs, and whole grains or spaghetti squash instead of white pastas and flours—sensible substitutions, not only for the weight benefit, but for the health benefit. And I learned about portion control.

Before, when I'd eat cereal, I thought I was making a healthy choice, even though I was eating two full cups! One time, I had been craving cheesecake for a week, and I knew if I put it off any longer I'd go to The Cheesecake Factory for a massive slice. Instead, I went to a small restaurant and had a garden salad with balsamic vinegar. For dessert, I had a little piece of crustless cheesecake. I've learned that if you deprive yourself, you'll eventually overindulge.

## MY FITNESS

I quickly discovered that I'm not a gym person, so I had to find other ways to exercise that I didn't hate. I started with Pilates, tried belly-dancing classes with friends, and eventually fell in love with Zumba. My boyfriend is now teaching me how to play tennis. I found activities that were more stimulating to me, and I try to exercise about four times a week. I also started walking more—I walk pretty much everywhere. I'm more active now, and I'm probably more outgoing as well. When you're not happy, people pick up on it. Now people notice how happy I am.

## MY PAYOFF

When I reached my goal weight, I was in disbelief. I never thought it would happen. I cried! It's such a relief to know I'm finally healthy. Having my family's support has been invaluable. I had told everyone I was doing Weight Watchers, which helped me stick with it when I had a setback—I had to save face! After my mom and I joined, my sister joined as well, and then my aunt and uncle in Arizona joined, plus my cousin and his girlfriend in Orlando. My mom's back at her goal weight, my sister lost 40 pounds, and my aunt and uncle have reached their goals. My dad even lost 50 pounds, just because of my mom's healthy food!

# {CHAPTER 6}
# Sweat—
## A Love Story

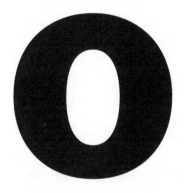F ALL OF THE TRANSFOR-
MATIVE, life-changing habits
I have developed since my start
with Weight Watchers, none
is more important to me than
exercise. Fitness has elevated
my quality of life and who I am.
Hubris? Definitely not.

First off, why does exercise
matter? My view has always
been that I could never have lost weight by exercise alone. It is
also my strong belief that I never would have kept my weight
off without exercise. Working out smooths over many sins in
the often bumpy road of maintenance. After all, a regular and
reasonably intense bout of exercise can create about a 300
calorie buffer per day. And working out and building muscle is
a great way to offset any potential drops in metabolism resulting from weight loss.

The National Weight Control Registry, a long-term research
study that tracks 10,000 adults who've lost at least 30 pounds,
notes that 90 percent of its successful weight loss maintainers
practice a combination of good nutrition and regular exercise.
Frankly, it's pretty hard to win at the healthy lifestyle game by
sprinting down to the Shake Shack for a large fries. You've got
to earn it at the table and burn it at the gym.

There are two kinds of exercise, and they both play an important role in health and weight maintenance.

- **Cardiovascular:** In its Physical Activity Guidelines for Americans, the US Department of Health and Human Services recommends at least 150 minutes per week (2.5 hours) of moderate intensity aerobic activity for health. It actively encourages 300 minutes of moderate activity (5 hours) to go beyond health benefits like lowering blood pressure and improving sleep. So you'll need to make more than a minimum effort to enjoy benefits like weight management and a stronger heart.

- **Strength training:** Those same guidelines also encourage 2 hours of strength training per week. The value of strength training is wide ranging. One simple way to think about it is that as you build muscle, you not only look more shapely, you burn calories during the workout and for up to 24 hours afterward. Muscle is the key driver in metabolism.

In sum, then: Cardiovascular exercise burns calories while you are on the run, while strength training helps burn them during exercise and while you are resting afterward. Kind of a nice one-two punch.

The logic of fully embracing the level of exercise recommended by the guidelines is: (1) it's good for your health, (2) it helps you manage your weight, and (3) it makes your birthday suit fit better. All three of these are obviously appealing, but how does one go from athletic zero to hero? For many, the thought of regular exercise is pretty daunting. This was absolutely the case for me.

# Finding My Inner Athlete

When I meet people today, many of them speculate that I have been an athlete all my life. They ask what sports I played in college, and they presume that exercise has been a permanent fixture in my life. I'm grateful for the implied compliments, but the notion that I was a jock from age 7 could not be further from the truth.

As a youngster, I was a boy colt: all arms and legs and little knowledge how to move them around. My eye-hand coordination was horrific. My elementary school gym teachers held me in bitter contempt, and I don't blame them. Yeah, I felt bad for me, too, thanks.

I grew into my skin a little in my teens, but I was still not ready for Division I sports. I wasn't graceful enough for finesse roles but still too skinny to fend off an offensive lineman. I accepted that I would have to find other outlets.

During these early years, I had my first romance with a sport: biking. My father gave me his 10-speed racing bike, which was not getting much use. It was an Italian bike, equipped with nifty Campagnolo gear, which I thought was pretty fancy. I started to ride regularly and became a bit

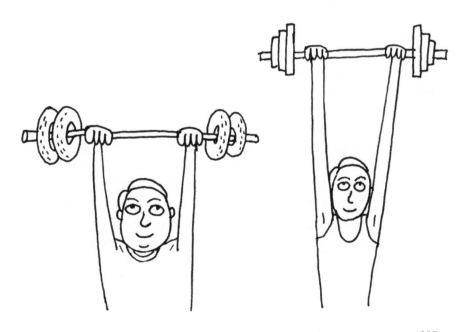

of a bicycle geek. I loved the process of disassembling and reassembling my bike. I also began to love riding it. It was the first time I ever realized the power of exercise to expand my horizons and to make me feel better and more alive.

In college, I became friends with the weight room, where most of my friends were grunting and sweating. In my mind, it was what dudes did, so I was happy to stick with it. I started to adopt a more rounded fitness routine, and I even tried out running.

For my first few years out of college, my job did not require a lot of travel, so I could keep up with my gym schedule. At the time, I was hitting the weight room probably twice a week. By the time I turned 25, I had gotten myself respectably strong, and fitness had become a habit.

Except then it wasn't. In 1991, I was off to Chicago and business school and, from there, management consulting. All of a sudden I was traveling constantly, so I pretty much stopped exercising. I would hit the gym maybe five or six times a month. The only exercise left in my schedule was going for walks with my wife on weekends. I became a sloth—the five-toed variety. I basically blew off exercise for the better part of 6 years.

Then my life got better and much worse at the same time. The "better" part: I started as an employee of Weight Watchers.com, Inc. at the end of January 2000, and on February 29, 2000, we had our second baby girl, Lila. Our house went into free-time lockdown. Having a newborn and a 2-year-old, separated by 2 years and 2 days, the parental units kicked into overdrive. Sleep became a distant memory for me and my wife. Neither of us had a moment to ourselves.

Within a couple of months, I made a remarkable discovery: an unused scattering of exercise equipment in the basement. Sure, I'd bought the dumbbells, a bench, and an exercise bike, but they were just more junk in our basement. Soon after Lila was born, however, I found myself desperately seeking some "me" time. I went down to the basement with a boom box, a mix tape, and a desire to work out my stress. I lifted weights for the first time in too many years, and I kind of liked it. The next day, I bought a book on weight lifting routines and cobbled together my own homegrown lifting regimen. I started to work out early in the morning a couple of days a week.

For me, the trigger wasn't better health or bulging muscles, but rather, the freedom to listen to music in the solitude of my basement. It doesn't take much really, does it? Over time, I started to build a routine that included setting out my gym clothes at night so I wouldn't have a good excuse to fall back asleep when the alarm went off.

This was great for a while. The only issue with my basement workout routine was that it felt kind of creepy. The basement in our house bore a striking resemblance to the one in *Silence of the Lambs* where the guy bred butterflies. It was just a little too serial-killer-esque, so I abandoned my workout buddy Hannibal and joined a gym.

I enjoy good gear, so I loved the gym's squat racks, plus other cool medieval torture devices that I never would have bought for myself. The other advantage was that I liked the social aspect of it. I found being around others energizing. To this day, I get a kick out of seeing the 5 a.m. workout people outside the gym. We always recognize each other with a smile, knowing that we are members of the tribe of freaky exercise people, even if we don't know one another's names.

Today, I lift weights 4 days a week, using a strategy called splits to work two areas of my body each day (see "4-Day Fitness" on page 128). I do this week in and week out so I never let myself off the hook. I should probably change up my routine more and "shock" my muscles, which some exercise physiologists claim brings faster results and averts a plateau. While I intellectually understand this, my workout routines have become fairly autopilot, which is a good thing for me. Others need variety in their exercise. I need to keep my muscles on autopilot, or they just might crash into the empty weekend.

*(continued on page 130)*

# 4-Day Fitness

Over the years, I kept at my weight lifting. I started doing what bodybuilders call a split routine, in which I would exercise different muscle groups on different days of the week. You exhaust one muscle group, then give it a rest while you work on another part of your body. This is a balanced way of building all-over tone.

Eventually I settled into a 4-day split, which goes as follows:

**DAY 1**

## Legs and abdominals

- 4 sets of squats (free bar)
- 4 sets of leg presses (sled)
- 3 sets of calf raises
- 3 sets of leg extensions (machine)
- 3 sets of hamstring curls (machine)
- 3 sets of hip abductors (machine)
- 3 sets of hip adductors (machine)
- 4 abdominal exercises (various), 3 sets each

**DAY 2**

## Back and biceps

- 3 sets of wide grip pullups
- 3 sets of chinups
- 3 sets of roman back extensions (machine)
- 3 sets of dumbbell rows
- 3 sets of dumbbell shrugs
- 3 sets of curls (E-Z Curl Bar)
- 3 sets of concentration curls
- 3 sets of wrist curls
- 3 sets of hammer curls (dumbbell)
- 3 sets of reverse wrist curls

## DAY 3
# Chest and triceps

- 3 sets of flat bench presses (bar)
- 3 sets of incline bench presses (bar)
- 3 sets of decline bench presses (bar)
- 3 sets of dumbbell flies
- 3 sets of triceps skull crushers
- 3 sets of triceps push-downs (cable)
- 3 sets of seated triceps extensions (dumbbell)

## DAY 4
# Shoulders and abdominals

- 3 sets of shoulder presses (Smith machine)
- 3 sets of behind the neck military presses (Smith machine)
- 3 sets of close grip upright rows (Smith machine)
- 3 sets of shoulder raises (dumbbell)
- 3 sets of lateral raises (dumbbell)
- 4 abdominal exercises (various), 3 sets each

For compulsive people like me, the split routine is beautiful. I cannot skip any of the 4 days or else the Earth would cease to spin on its axis. Accordingly, I have probably had 10 weeks in the past 250 in which I did not do all 4 days. I was able to create my own routine without help, but I have seen trainers help many people get into and adopt weight lifting into their daily lives.

Ultimately, for me the most fun aspect to weight lifting has been getting stronger. It embarrasses me a little to admit that I love the fact that I can bench-press more today than I could at any other point in my life. It's an empowering feeling, like going from the Barcalounger to the marathon finish line over a period of years.

And that brings me to my cardio workouts. I had felt that I'd probably gone as far as I was likely to go in building in new weight lifting exercises into my routine. I wanted to open up my exercise to a new level, so I finally added cardio to my week. I chose the bicycle, in its many forms, as my route in. Biking felt like a good way to get my heart moving while remaining fairly low impact on my aging body. I started with a couple of days a week on the stationary bike. Then I discovered the pain and glory of Spinning classes. Finally, I went out and bought my first new road bike in more than 20 years. I was a kid on my dad's Italian bike once again.

My first year getting back on my bike was exercise, all right— an exercise in humility. I would slog up hills and get to the top a heaving mess, clocking about 7 mph in an embarrassingly low granny gear. But just as with weight lifting, I knew that if I stuck with it, I would build endurance. Sure enough I did, and I was able to tackle hills with enough energy to keep up with my chain-gang friends. I now count my road bike as one of my very best fitness buddies.

Now I was a cardio exercise guy as well as a gym rat.

These days, I exercise 6 to 7 days per week, and I'm proud of that fact. I'm especially proud because I most certainly did not start this way. I am hardly unique. I have met lots of people who went from sedentary slacker to marathon finisher. What all of us new exercisers have in common is that we gradually worked our way into it. You can, too. It's never too late to become an athlete.

So what have I learned on my 8-year road to regular exercise?

# 1. IT'S ALL ABOUT THE ROUTINE

For me, regular exercise, like diet, is not about discipline or heroic willpower—it's much more about routine. Regular exercise becomes ingrained when you develop new habits that ultimately become a way of life.

One of my big tricks in exercising was to create a set of conditions that would take away every reason to blow off the gym and fall back to sleep. My morning ritual:

- I set out my gym clothes by the computer in our office the night before. My logic for this is that my good intentions are running high before I go to bed, so I'm happy to perform this proactive step. I don't want to have to rely on any good intentions whatsoever when the alarm goes off at 5 a.m.

- I also set out a Sugar Free Red Bull next to the mouse pad of my computer. I know I am setting a bad example with my energy drinks, but grant a man a few vices, please. I know that early-morning boost of caffeine and other unknown chemicals will help give me a little push.

- I never hit snooze when the alarm goes off. I immediately leave the bed and hit my home office as quickly as possible. The last thing I need is a debate about whether I'd like to sleep some more. It's an argument the bed would win every time, so I just skip that step.

- I check my e-mail, the news, and the weather, and I am off to the gym by 5:30 a.m.

If I do this morning ritual plus my 4-day split plus scheduled Spinning classes, I really do not make any decisions whatsoever. I do not use my brain at all. I just go and do. This is not discipline, this is a mindless habit. It just happens to be mindlessly good for me.

Now my exercise habit is so strong that I become agitated if I cannot work out. It's my default state, but reaching this place did not happen overnight. It took time.

# 2. ARRANGE YOUR OWN "BIG BOWL OF CHEESE"

Over time, I have found exercise to be its own reward. But in those early days, I needed something to look forward to—immediate gratification the second I entered the gym.

Loud music!

It was Saturday morning. I had not slept well the previous night, tossing and turning from 4 a.m. on. My head hurt, I was unmotivated and generally crabby. Not a pretty sight. I needed a fix.

In years past, a gargantuan breakfast burrito (chorizo, queso, many eggs, lots of grease) served with a side of home fries and an English muffin (slathered with butter and jam) would have fixed me up quickly. The comforting effects of fat should never be underestimated. This was exactly the remedy that the completely understanding devil perched on my left shoulder was whispering in my ear. But the preachy angel on my right shoulder was exhorting me to take the hard but rewarding turn at the fork in the road. "Work out!" he said. "You will feel much better after a good sweat!"

I was not in the mood to hear it. But I steeled myself to take the righteous path. I was filled with dread as I went to the gym, thinking about the stationary bike awaiting me. I needed a good 45 minutes of exercise-induced pain, and this bike would deliver. Was I up to it? I pulled out my secret weapon: a mix of cheesy, big, loud music. In fact, I named this playlist the "Giant Bowl of Cheese." It worked. I finished my 45 minutes with a self-satisfied smile on my face.

I have relied on music for motivational breakthrough more times than I can count.

Working out to good tunes is hardly a new concept. Richard Simmons broke historic ground with *Sweatin' to the Oldies,* and life hasn't been the same since. Everybody in the gym wears earphones, and Richard deserves full credit.

My personal trick is to employ a battery of music that I might be a little bashful about listening to without headphones.

The sampling that Saturday included: Rush, Guns N' Roses, Asia, Journey, Steve Miller, and the massively motivating Bee Gees. This stuff works magic on me. I've never had a bad 4-minute exercise stretch with "Staying Alive" blaring through my earbuds. The other trick is to have enough on the mix so I can shuffle it and never get bored. These days, I have about 10 to 12 go-to albums plus another 7 to 8 playlists that I use to keep things interesting. iTunes has been a wonderful workout motivator.

If you give loud, cheesy workout soundtracks a go, please consider two important safety tips:

• Excessively loud music combined with earbuds equals deafness. Say what?

• Public air guitaring is not acceptable, especially on a stationary bike. You could hurt someone that way.

# 3. PREWIRE YOUR DAY FOR EXERCISE NO MATTER WHERE YOU ARE

In a prior life, being out of town or on vacation would have been reason enough to blow off a workout. Now I make space in my life for exercise. This means planning ahead, and even scheduling it into my calendar if need be.

Equinox fitness club is near my office at work, and there's one in my hometown. I belong to both, so there goes another excuse: It's always convenient to pop in for a workout. I know where everything is, and I build my workout routine around their standard setups. As noted, I take comfort in the familiar. I advise you to belong to a gym that's so close you trip over it on your way to and from work, shopping, whatever.

If you're a runner or a walker, so much the better. Your workout can be anywhere, and that's a big advantage. My beloved Equinox isn't everywhere, but gyms are in fact as ubiquitous as Dunkin' Donuts and McDonald's (ironic). Here are my tricks for staying in the game when I'm on the road:

• **VACATION STRATEGY:** I scout out a gym ahead of time. Most vacation spots have local gyms that are more than happy to sell a 1-to-2-week temporary membership. This has worked on virtually every vacation I have ever taken within the United States—it's a little trickier outside the country.

• **HOTEL STRATEGY #1:** I stay at hotels that have full-service gyms. Every full-service hotel will say it has a fitness center. Usually, *fitness center* is French for "four pieces of crummy equipment." Not as good as a real gym, but they will do in a pinch.

• **HOTEL STRATEGY #2:** Stay at a hotel that's close to a full-service gym. I did this recently in San Diego, and the hotel was able to sell me a $15 pass for the local 24 Hour Fitness. It was a great gym, and it made me smile. I've used the local gym strategy not only in the United States, but also in Europe (London, Paris, Barcelona, Düsseldorf) and Australia.

When it comes to living a healthier life, a little research and advanced planning can take you a long way and make you feel more at home.

# 4. EVERY ONCE IN A WHILE, TRY SOMETHING NEW (DO AS I SAY, NOT AS I DO)

Yes, I'm a creature of workout habit. But if you really want the best results from your exercise—the greatest boost to your calorie burn, strength, and stamina—it pays to surprise your muscles with new routines and challenges. You can achieve that by trying novel classes, changing sports with the seasons, or even just building new exercises, pacing, or weights into old workouts. The rule of thumb is: If you do the same thing every day, you'll achieve the same results every day. Your body will literally stop responding. To improve, move from one thing to another to another.

For my own workouts, I'm pretty much of a lone wolf (dark

and mysterious, even). My weight lifting routine is too much of a Rube Goldberg device to expect others to do it with me or to find room for a personal trainer in my complicated mix. When it comes to cardio, I am also an individual player, preferring to jack in my own tunes on a Lifecycle and attack it at my own pace.

Still, I have occasionally tried communal sporting endeavors. For instance: Spinning.

My first brush with Spinning was at my local Equinox. Immediately, I saw that solo cycling was no match for it. I would find myself pushing at least 50 to 75 percent harder in Spinning class than when pedaling on my own. I've been wondering why this is the case. My theory:

- **The Spinning instructor:** She (Emma) seems like a nice, kind, decent person—until she swings into the saddle of a bike. That's when she becomes dictatorial and a little bit abusive.

  "David, you're spinning too fast, you need more resistance!"

  "I need you to get to a place where you are kind of miserable."

  "You should be feeling nasty by now."

  This is not nice behavior, but it works. When someone looks you in the eye and tells you to push harder, you do.

- **Peer pressure:** When I exercise on my own, I feel like a stud. In my solo-workout mind, I'm pushing my pedals harder than what anyone has ever attempted before. I rule! In a Spinning class, I see everyone keeping pace while jacking up the tension on their spinning wheel. I stink. Therefore I push to keep up. (I cannot rule out the possibility that they're just pretending to jack up the tension on their wheel. Not that I would ever do this.)

Bottom line: My desire for the approval of others and my inherent competitiveness make this format pretty ideal, even if it reduces me to a sweaty, heaving mess.

I've also surrendered to the trendoids and tried yoga. I have historically been pretty skeptical about the whole spiritual exercise thing. I prefer the route of the knuckle dragger, clinging to my free weights. However, I decided to give yoga a try for two reasons:

- **Stretching:** I am probably the least flexible person I know. It's a little sad that someone who considers himself to be in really good shape cannot touch his toes without a sizable knee bend. I saw yoga as a way to get in a huge range of stretching that I would otherwise never do.

- **Getting my Zen on:** My brain feels like it's in constant overdrive, barreling from thought to thought without ever cruising down the off-ramp. Meditation is a great way to settle the brain and improve concentration.

Ultimately, I was not able to make the yoga routine stick. Yoga classes can take 90 minutes start to finish, and I simply could not find the time to work in the additional commitment. Becoming a yoga person would have required me to be flexible on my 4-day weight lifting split, and that was more than I could bear. I would never rule out yoga for the future, but for now I'm sticking with the knuckle draggers.

This leads to insight #5 . . .

# 5. FIND SOMETHING YOU CAN LOVE (AT LEAST A LITTLE BIT)

Just because the cool kids are doing yoga is not reason enough to join them. The exercises I do are the ones I like to do.

An old friend gave me a copy of *What I Talk About When I Talk About Running* by Haruki Murakami. Murakami is a prolific Japanese novelist who, at the age of 33, sold his jazz bar in Japan and ditched cigarettes. He went on to be a marathon runner and a triathlete. It is a wonderful, spiritual book about the transformative and meditative effects of running.

I loved the book, and I hate running. To that point, I always remind myself of Murakami's observation that runners love to run. Either you find that spark or you do not. He found his later in life. My take is that either you find a way to fall in love with an exercise or you don't. I suppose exercise is like mating. You have to keep trying until you find the one you can fall in love with.

I would never fall in love with running, but I did fall pretty hard for the weight room. Over the past few years, I have also found myself getting romantic with my bicycle again. What can I say? I'm kind of an exercise harlot.

# 6. CONSIDER MEASURING

Once I suspected that not all cycling activities are created equal, I became obsessed with measuring each of them. To figure it out, I bought a Garmin heart rate monitor (the FR60, for those who are shopping—I like it!).

A heart rate monitor, for the uninitiated, measures the intensity of an activity measured by heartbeats per minute compared to a maximum heart rate based on age (you can find out more by looking at those Physical Activity Guidelines for Americans on line).

In no time, I discovered that the Spinning class literally torched me, cranking my heart rate up to 85 percent of my maximum compared with 81 percent of my maximum on a road bike (not bad—and I tended to ride longer when outdoors) and just 77 percent on a Lifecycle. You can use a heart rate monitor for any cardio activity, to keep pushing yourself harder and to make sure you take adequate amounts of rest. They typically come with detailed instructions for use, and now even connect to your computer to download and track your results.

My conclusions from my heart-rate monitor experiment:

- **Accept punishment from a teacher:** The effect of having my good friend Emma (the Spinning instructor from the depths of Hades) hammering on me works out to about a 9 percent increase in average heart rate versus the Lifecycle.

- **Duration counts:** The road bike trip was the calorie-inferno winner. I put in 62 percent more minutes on my bike than I did on the Lifecycle, yet my average heart rate was still 5 percent higher.

- **Time to man-up on the stationary bike:** I need to up the average resistance on the Lifecycle. Points #1 and #2 clearly demonstrate that I could push myself harder.

My other conclusions are that, yes, I am truly a geek for spending this much time analyzing all of this stuff. Second, the old adage of "what gets measured gets done" is true. The heart rate monitor helped me take my exercise to the next level. I needed that.

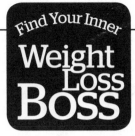

## If food is the key to weight loss, exercise is the fudge factor. (It allows you to burn off indiscretions.) Now make it stick.

### Start slow, but start with full intention.

I have never met anyone who went from zero exercise to running a marathon in 2 months. I have met lots of people who started walking, moved on to 5-Ks, made it to marathons, and, in some cases, did triathlons. For me, one of the most rewarding parts of exercise has been how I have been able to build it up over time. It makes looking back at the distance I have come all the more rewarding.

### Find something you love.

People embrace exercise in so many different ways. Some live for their yoga, while others love to run. Some love their group exercise, while others like to go for long solo walks. Weight lifting and biking became my things. They work for me. Find what works for you.

### Measure what you do.

Countless studies show how people tend to overestimate how much they exercise. Consider stepping up to a pedometer, heart rate monitor, or accelerometer. It's a great way to find out how much you are actually moving. This can help you fine-tune your calorie intake, but it's also a great way of setting new goals and challenging yourself to push harder.

### Most important: Make exercise a priority.

Lots of people talk about their desire to exercise more, but they just cannot find the time for it. What if exercise was as important as eating? Would we find time for it then? I became an early-morning workout person because I knew I would always have time for it at that hour. Schedule it into your life and protect it on your calendar. Stop thinking of exercise as a nice-to-have and start treating it as a need-to-have.

## Weight Watchers Profile

### "If I plan to be successful, I will be successful."

Hard work, determination, and discipline pay off.

**Ann Farrankop, 43,**
*Redwood City, CA*

**HEIGHT:** 5 feet 2 inches
**WEIGHT BEFORE:** 221
**WEIGHT AFTER:** 118
Reached her goal in 15 months

### MY STRUGGLE

My job requires me to be on my feet all day. So when I'd leave work, I would just sit on the couch and watch TV while I ate. The inactivity did me in. Plus, my portions were out of control. I was eating too much. I was working too much. I found myself trapped in the yo-yo cycle, and I was miserable.

### MY WAKE-UP CALL

I was at the park playground babysitting my niece, and she landed on my knee. It shouldn't have hurt, but it did. A couple of minutes later, I couldn't walk. Being in so much pain forced me to rethink my weight and what I was doing to my body. I figured that if I could take that extra weight out of the equation, I'd be healthier—and happier.

### MY FOOD

It took me a while to learn that too much of a good thing is not a good thing. I grew up eating my mom's homemade meals—if her lasagna was in front of me, I could eat the whole pan. Now I weigh and measure all of my food and write down what I eat in a journal every day. Sometimes it's tedious, but losing the weight makes it worth the extra effort. I know that if I plan to be successful, then I will be successful.

## MY FITNESS

I hit the gym at least 5 days per week and work with a trainer twice a week. I log 30 minutes of cardio on the elliptical machine and perform mat exercises to strengthen my core. Outside the gym, I wear a pedometer to measure how much I'm walking and try to take extra steps whenever I can.

## MY PAYOFF

I fit into a size 4! Every day I look in the mirror at what I've achieved. I have a motto tacked on my wall that says, "Stand up and finish what you started." I'm so satisfied every day, knowing I finished what I started. I'm thinner now than I've ever been. My body is transforming. I'm becoming muscular. My legs and arms are transforming. My self-esteem is back—and my knee pain is gone. The hard work, determination, and discipline pay off.

# {CHAPTER 7}

# The Change-Your-Lifestyle Tool Kit

## Your New Utility Belt

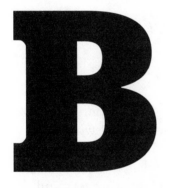

**B**ATMAN WAS ULTIMATELY A SUPERHERO because of Bruce Wayne. His superhero-ness came from who Bruce was within. It came from his character. It came from his desire to achieve by fighting guys with bad makeup. Batman also had a sweet utility belt and an even sweeter bat car. Those gadgets didn't make him a superhero, but they most definitely helped. Everyone has the ability to achieve great things and become the boss of their weight loss—or weight loss superhero, if you will. That said, we could all use a nice utility belt to help us succeed.

In making all of the changes discussed in the previous chapters, and in facing the many challenges in front of us, we should all seek to employ the right set of tools to help us be more mindful, stay on track, stay motivated, and stay successful. Simply put, it's easier to lose weight and achieve a healthier lifestyle with a little help.

My personal Batman kit was provided by the nice folks at Weight Watchers, but it's certainly not the only way to go. In this chapter, I will talk about Weight Watchers, but mostly so I can illustrate how a set of basic tools and support systems helped me. I cannot recommend my own company enough, but there are other places you can also find support. I'm just not going to tell you where—I'm way too competitive to do that. Also, the tools below are the ones that had the biggest impact for me in my success, and they are the same ones that are routinely referenced by lots of smart people in the field of weight loss. Therefore, do not think of this list as exhaustive, but rather consider each tool and think of how it can help, not how it might enslave you.

# A Utility Belt to Cinch Around Your Shrinking Waist

When people say nice things about Weight Watchers, they often use phrases such as "It's the only thing that works" and "It just makes sense." Even better, I hear people say that Weight Watchers is not a diet, it's a lifestyle.

When people distinguish between Weight Watchers and dieting, they're reflecting the negative connotation of the term *diet*. In popular parlance, a diet is often seen as an unnatural act that one does for a period of 2 months to get ready for a beach vacation/wedding/reunion/divorce. After the big event, the dieter returns to real life.

But a lifestyle is a way of living and making choices in the world. A new healthy lifestyle is harder to pull off, but it is ultimately the only path you can sustain. In fact, Weight Watchers is in the sustained-gains business. We give people the system, tools, and support to help them create their own healthy lifestyles.

When I meet someone who has had great success on our program, he or she will often thank me/us for changing his or her life. I always say the same thing to these people: Your success is completely yours. I'm just glad we could help.

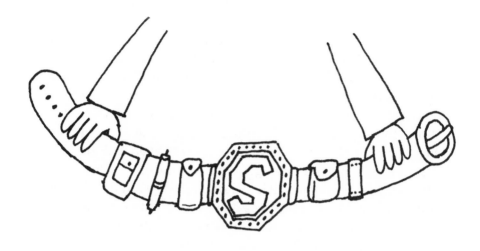

I really do believe it. Weight Watchers is not a magic system for miracle weight loss. The only way anybody can lose weight is to make different choices and live in a different way. The sooner that you put your belief and trust in yourself, the sooner you will realize that you manage own destiny. When you reach that point, you will seek the tools and support that help you achieve your own goals and dreams.

Not my goals. Not Weight Watchers' goals. Your own.

When people ask me what Weight Watchers does, I roll out our mantra: We provide education and behavior change tools in a supportive environment to help people lose weight sustainably. That's a mouthful, I realize. In a clinical environment, we are referred to as a "community-based intensive multicomponent behavioral treatment provider." This is not a very sexy way of putting it, but it's a powerful statement about what we do.

Most of us have tried to lose weight on our own. We feel that if only we were stronger or more disciplined, then we never would have had a weight problem in the first place. We also blame ourselves for the weakness that caused the weight problem, and we seek a counterbalancing strength to muscle it away. We want to punish ourselves to succeed, in response to our self-doubt and regret.

In truth, changing behavior and creating new habits is not easy. It's even harder in a food environment that conspires against us. Frankly, we need all the help we can get to protect ourselves from the food peddlers, to keep us focused on the fight against mindless eating. That's why study after study shows that people have more success when they lose weight with the help of others than when they try to go it alone.

And it's not just me saying it. The *Journal of the American Medical Association* published a study in 2003 in which obese volunteers were randomly assigned to one of two groups: one group attended Weight Watchers; the other tried to lose weight on their own. Researchers followed them for 2 years. The results: Those attending Weight Watchers meetings lost, and kept off, three times more weight. The more meetings volunteers attended, the more weight they lost.

I'm not arguing that you need to become a member. Honestly. But there are certain tools and strategies that our company employs precisely because they are proven to work, and they are powerful. I want to share some of them with you here—namely, the ones that worked for me. They were the various gizmos on my Batman utility belt. Without them, I would not have gotten where I am today.

# Tracking

Some people think of the process of tracking as a form of dieting. I disagree. It's true that to lose weight, you need to reduce calorie intake. Keeping track of what you eat helps you do that. In my mind, tracking isn't a dieting activity per se. I think of it as training.

Imagine a friend who is bordering on bankruptcy, whose credit cards are maxed out, who is a shopaholic, and who seems out of control with money. The first advice you'd give that friend would be to make a budget. Then you'd suggest that he keep track of where he spends his money. Once he knows that, he could start making different choices—spending on priorities, saving on frivolities. It would be common sense.

Food takes this problem to the next level. We are constantly being reminded of how much things cost via price tags, receipts, and bank statements. With food, we have only a fleeting and often mistaken idea of what we are "spending" on energy intake. Nutrition scientists have shown that people underestimate how much they eat by about 30 percent, and they overestimate how much they exercise by 30 percent. That's the official definition of bad math.

Weight Watchers uses currency-based tracking methodology that keeps track of energy intake and energy output. For years, our original Points system (introduced in late 1997 in the United States) was based principally on calories, with a penalty for fat and a bonus for fiber. By late 2010, there had been major advances in nutrition science, so we revamped the currency system. We took the major macronutrient components of calories—protein, fats, carbohydrates, and fiber—and we performed a separate calculation on each one. These calculations measured gross energy, but they also took into consideration how hard the body had to work to convert the macronutrient components into useful energy. We also considered satiety.

In the new PointsPlus system, protein and fiber were treated more favorably, while carbs and fats were treated less favorably. We went a little further by ascribing zero PointsPlus values to most fruits and nonstarchy vegetables. In this new system, healthy whole foods went on sale while junk food and heavily processed foods got a lot more expensive.

So what useful purpose does tracking calories serve in a weight loss context?

# 1. EDUCATION: BETTER CHOICES, WORSE CHOICES

One of the often fun—and many times scary—parts of tracking is learning whether certain foods are good friends or sneaky assassins. I sometimes amuse myself by trying to find the most horribly high PointsPlus value foods around. Let's start with how tracking helps me navigate Panera Bread.

Were I not informed, I might not know that Panera's:

- Pumpkin muffin has 16 PointsPlus values (590 calories)

- Cinnamon chip scone has 17 PointsPlus values (610 calories)

- Sierra Turkey on Focaccia with Asiago Cheese has 25 PointsPlus values (920 calories)

- Fuji apple with chicken salad and ranch dressing has 19 PointsPlus vaues (700 calories)

Equipped with a PointsPlus calculator, you can make smarter choices from Panera's menu.

- A breakfast power sandwich has 9 PointsPlus values (340 calories).

- A smoked turkey breast on country bread will cost you just 11 PointsPlus values (420 calories).

- A full Greek salad with Thai Chili dressing has 12 PointsPlus values (430 calories).

For fun, one can always play "find the nastiest food on the menu" game. Some prime finds one might stumble upon could include:

- The Jack Daniels Ribs and Shrimp at T.G.I. Fridays clocks in at 47 PointsPlus values (1,740 calories).

- At Dairy Queen, the six-piece chicken tenders with country gravy will cost you 32 PointsPlus values (1,370 calories).

• A Dairy Queen large Chocolate Xtreme blizzard has 39 PointsPlus values (1,420 calories).

• A Five Guys bacon cheeseburger and large fries (plus a Diet Coke) breaks the food bank at 64 PointsPlus values (2,394 calories).

I could go on.

To put this all in perspective, I'm allotted around 40 PointsPlus values per day, and I'm a tall guy who's trying to maintain my weight. For many Weight Watchers members, that Five Guys feast would cost more than 2 days' worth of PointsPlus values. Better invite five guys along to help you eat it.

Tracking becomes even more helpful in clarifying the effect of portion sizes on our waist sizes. Portion distortion has become a huge issue in the world we live in today. We are truly living in a supersize world. Food companies and restaurants have tried to make us "happy" by giving us great value. The bigger the serving, the less we pay per ounce of food. Heaping portions may be cheap, but they are costly for our health.

Again, you don't have to rely on our system—you can track calories, fat, and energy density using any number of available books or apps designed to help you do that. Knowledge is power!

# 2. MINDFULNESS: THE POWER OF PAYING ATTENTION

It amazes me how much we eat without even realizing it. Grab a handful of nuts here, a few "harmless" candies there, another few chips, and it suddenly starts to add up. We tend to downplay these little moments, saying they don't count (especially if we purposely fail to do the math). But calories behave in the same way whether we're paying attention or not.

Tracking gives visibility to these hidden little food sneaks and sleights of hand. The old Weight Watchers maxim is "If you bite it, write it." This may sound a little obsessive, but it is a very effective way of making ourselves much more mindful of what we are doing and what we are chewing. In

Chapter 5, I talked about creating interventions to disrupt bad habits. Tracking is a great example of this.

# 3. BUDGETING: COST-EFFECTIVE CONSUMPTION

Research has shown pretty consistently that people who track calories and weight as they try to shed pounds have considerably more success than those who do not. It makes sense. If we have to live on less money, we reevaluate all of our spending decisions. If you're used to living on 60 PointsPlus values per day and then have to cut back to 40, you would reconsider all of your meal and snack choices. You would learn to live within the new budget and create meaningful new habits.

What about me? I'll confess that I am not naturally wired to track or budget. I dislike to-do lists, and I take no great joy in balancing my checkbook. In fact, my wife has done the financial management of our household for nearly two decades, and I'm very grateful to her for it.

But when the need is great and my wife is unavailable, I'll do it. I know I couldn't have changed my habits if I hadn't forced myself to track. My history with it has changed over the past 10 years as I have moved along the nutritional and behavior learning curve. For instance, I use tracking very differently today than I did when I first got started. It has played a number of different and important roles for me in my efforts to reform my eating and exercise habits.

## Early Years (2000 to 2003-ish)

The day I first started tracking Points values was a smack upside the head. Everything I thought I knew about the foods I ate was wrong, and every day I tracked was an education. Portion size was also a big revelation for me when I started tracking. It was a rude awakening to find out that one entree of Chinese food might be too much for one person in one sitting.

Once I incorporated the Points System values in my tool belt, I began making food choices with knowledge and discipline. I credit it as the biggest reason I started losing weight and keeping it off.

# Final Weight Loss: 2007

I had lost a bunch of weight, and I was pretty consistently down 20 pounds from my peak of 240-plus. However, I was still about 15 pounds from where I really needed to be. I started the year with the tracker by my side (or on my computer, to be more specific), and I waged war on ignorant eating. I redid my breakfast and lunch routines once and for all, with full knowledge of my Points values each day. I significantly reduced between-meal foraging (at least before dinner), and I jacked up my Activity Points values. Finally, I reached my goal weight, became a Lifetime Member, and entered into maintenance.

That I was at my target weight at all was largely due to tracking.

# Maintenance: 2007 to Present

It's now been close to 12 years from the first time I started tracking Points (now PointsPlus) values. I no longer track on a regular basis because I eat the same things for breakfast and for lunch, and I keep snacking to a minimum. At dinner, my wife is even better than tracking, because she controls my intake responsibly and deliciously.

So, have I now moved beyond tracking? No, but I use it in very specific ways.

**1. Course correction:** Sometimes after multiple weeks of travel or an aggressive social schedule, I can feel my better lifestyle start to slip away. If I ignore that this is happening, then I will start gaining weight. I can feel the landslide coming. At that point I pull out my iPhone and start tracking right away. It gets my head back into the game, and it refocuses me on applying reasonable restraint.

**2. Redirection:** I have a basket of Weight Watchers mini-bars outside my office. They are for visitors and to encourage colleagues who might otherwise be afraid of me to at least walk by my office. There are times when I consider plowing through three to four of those little guys myself. But I know that I will need to track these 4-second snacks, so I almost always divert myself to my refrigerator for a zero-PointsPlus value apple instead. My tracker is kind of like my security system, keeping me from breaking and entering the calorie vault.

**3. Attacking persistent weaknesses:** I can wander pretty far off the reservation on weekends. I still struggle with mindless munching after dinner, both at home and on the road. I also know that if I want to address these weak spots, I need a tool to help me. In this context, I have recently been focusing my tracking on weekend days and post-dinner. I know that if I make myself track what I eat, I will be much less likely to mindlessly munch. If I can keep this going, then I have a real shot at maintaining healthier habits.

# CONCLUSION

There are two ways I could look at tracking:

A tool enslaving me (i.e., the wrong way): This is the prison-term mentality. "Mr. Kirchhoff, the court has sentenced you to a lifetime of tracking with no hope of parole." Not guilty, your honor! Or . . .

A really awesome tool to help me achieve something bigger (the right way). Tracking, as a supercool tool, is very much like my iPhone or iPad. These are well-designed gadgets that make my life easier and help me to be more successful. The point is not the act of tracking itself. The point is establishing better and healthier habits. The tracker is simply the tool that makes me much more likely to do that. When I look at it this way, it's my personal assistant, not my master.

So, my last piece of advice is to take advantage of sweet tools. Having a giant Web site, a big collection of tools, and now an arsenal of iPhone applications has made the process of staying on track massively easier and more convenient.

Recently, Weight Watchers launched a bar code scanner application for the iPhone/Android. I just wave my phone over the bar code of grocery items, and it quickly tells me how many PointsPlus values are at play. While it's great fun and ridiculously convenient, I will admit to looking slightly odd when I shop, and I get giddy every time I find a calorie bargain.

On its most basic level, keeping a food diary is tracking. Regardless of whether you follow Weight Watchers or any other system, keeping track of what you eat is an important and powerful tool.

# Meet Your Friend, the Scale

Losing weight is a long road, and we need tools that allow us to stay on track, keep driving, and give us ways to measure our progress. After all of this time, the most basic way of doing this is still the scale. The point of using a scale is not to create obsession about how much you weigh or whether the number you see is accurate. Rather the point of the scale is to help you keep track of progress and to stay focused and motivated. Again, think of it as a behavior tool, not as the be-all and end-all.

Let's start with a basic review of metrics for keeping score.

## BMI

Body mass index, or BMI, expresses the relationship between weight and height, so it provides a more accurate measure than body weight alone.

The formula for calculating BMI is to divide a person's weight in kilograms by the square of his or her height in meters:

$$\text{BMI} = \frac{\text{Weight (kg)}}{\text{Height (m}^2).}$$

Online calculators that automatically do the computations are a convenient method of determining BMI. (There's a handy one on WeightWatchers.com.)

This particular measurement has some limitations. It tends to overestimate body fat in some people and underestimate it in others. BMI also doesn't show where the body fat is located. (Abdominal fat carries the greatest health risk.)

But at the end of the day, BMI is a good guide to knowing where you fit in the body-fat arena. More than 50 health care organizations around the world, including the US National Institutes of Health, use the same BMI standards to define adult overweight and obesity.

| DEFINITION | BMI |
| --- | --- |
| Overweight | 25–29.9 |
| Obese | 30–39.9 |
| Morbidly Obese | 40+ |

BMI is used as the standard to diagnose overweight and obesity because there are so many studies that show a link between BMI and the risk of many diseases and death.

As BMI increases, so does the risk for several conditions, including:

Diabetes

Cardiovascular disease

Stroke

Hypertension

Gallbladder disease

Osteoarthritis

Sleep apnea

Some cancers

Premature death

While the link between BMI and disease risk is clear, it is important to remember that it is only one of several disease risk factors. In other words, BMI cannot tell an individual that he or she will get a disease, only that the risk of developing the disease is increased.

# WAIST CIRCUMFERENCE

BMI is not the only indicator of weight-related health problems. The way that fat is distributed around the body also plays an important role. For example, body fat that accumulates around the waist, known as abdominal fat (an apple shape), poses a greater health risk than fat carried in the hips and thighs (a pear shape).

Men are genetically predisposed to gain weight around their waist, although there are exceptions. By contrast, women's bodies tend to be more pear shaped. Overweight men also tend to have more visceral fat, the fat that surrounds the organs in your middle, which substantially increases the risk of heart disease, metabolic syndrome, and diabetes.

Waist circumference has been studied extensively and is shown to be a reliable measure of abdominal fat—it's also an independent predictor of risk. A high waist circumference (greater than 35 inches in women and 40 inches in men) is linked to an increased risk for type 2 diabetes, dyslipidemia, hypertension, and heart disease.

How to measure waist circumference? While standing, locate your upper hip bone and place a tape measure around your waist (ensuring that the tape measure is horizontal). The tape measure should be snug but should not cause compressions on the skin.

Bottom line: You should know your BMI and waist circumference numbers. If they are not in the healthy range, it's time to take action and lose weight.

# BODY-WEIGHT COMPOSITION

Yet another way of keeping score is calculating body fat percentage. Simply stated, body-fat percentage is the weight of a person's body fat divided by their total weight. People who are very muscular and weigh a lot, but do not have excess fat, will have a low body fat percentage. Chances are they will also have a relatively low waist circumference. The advantage of tracking body fat percentage is pretty intuitive: It seems to directly measure the one variable that is of highest concern, fat.

### AVERAGE BODY FAT PERCENTAGES
(from the American Council on Exercise)

| CLASSIFICATION | WOMEN (% FAT) | MEN (% FAT) |
|---|---|---|
| Essential fat | 10–13% | 2–5% |
| Athletes | 14–20% | 6–13% |
| Fit | 21–24% | 14–17% |
| Average | 25–31% | 18–24% |
| Obese | 32%+ | 25%+ |

Body fat percentage is hard to measure accurately, and you typically need to consult a professional. The primary ways of measuring it that are available to folks like you and me include electric impedance (sending a current through the body to track how the jolt travels through fat layers), skin fold tests (done with icy cold calipers, in my experience), height and circumference measurements, and other methods. One can even go so far as to get a full water submersion test, which borders on Chinese water torture. The degree of accuracy can vary between all these methods, and that limits its use.

So before you dive into the water tank, it's helpful to be clear about why you're getting the measurement in the first place: (1) to gauge whether you are healthy, or (2) to measure your progress. Both objectives have their application. For the purpose of measuring regular progress, the scale has huge benefits. You can measure being down 1 pound, but that kind of change will not show up in your waist circumference.

# THE GOOD OLD SCALE

A pretty large battery of research shows that getting regular weigh-ins is a good predictor of sticking with a weight loss process and keeping the weight off once you've lost it. The National Weight Control Registry has found that people who are weighed regularly are much more likely to succeed. The long-term weight loss maintainers who were part of the registry's panel are vigilant about weight gain: If it pushes into the +5 percent range, they immediately redouble their efforts to get back on track.

Those of us who yo-yo between gains and losses too often tell ourselves that our weight is not really increasing, and we avoid the scale because we don't want to hear its testimony. After months of denial, we find we've regained much of our lost weight.

I regularly gauge where I am in my weight, principally by either getting a weigh-in or by checking how my pants fit. The scale doesn't lie, and the nature of the reckoning is motivating as well. I simply would not have stuck with the program if I was not being weighed regularly at Weight Watchers meetings. Period.

Don't I own a scale at home? Yes, I do. Do I know how to use it? Yes, I do. Am I capable of writing down the result? Yup. So why go someplace else and have someone do it for me?

Because the Weight Watchers scale brings powerful mojo into play. My inherent competitiveness, for one. And there is something about having someone else tell you to stand on a scale, write your weight down, and indicate whether you gained or lost. Having someone else bear witness to my success or failure is incredibly motivating, and it creates a moment of truth each week that cannot be dodged.

Consider my ritual before an official weigh-in. Let's say it is at 11 a.m. on a Thursday. I live like a monk the day(s) before. The morning of the weight-in, I often skip breakfast (not a good practice, I realize). I avoid drinking too many fluids, and I try to use the bathroom before the big moment. Before I step on the scale, I pull off my shoes and my watch, and ditch my wallet. Pockets: empty. Yes, when I dressed that morning I had considered whether I was wearing "heavy" clothes. As I get ready to stand on the scale, my stomach lurches into my throat, and I start sweating bullets (evaporative weight loss!). I know this makes me sound like an obsessed, crazy person, but having a good weigh-in really matters to me.

Frankly, I'm a little afraid of the scale. I fear that it might tell me I'm falling back on old habits. I'm afraid of defeat and having the scale can run up the "L" flag. Of course, this is a dumb way to react to an inanimate object. But it's the best way for me to know that I'm getting off track so I can quickly correct my course. It would be much worse for me to avoid the scale and then discover that I was up 20 pounds.

How should you use the scale? It's a little easy to overthink it, but my general advice is this: Be consistent and be regular. I like to weigh myself before lunch, but others hit the scale right after they get out of bed. It really doesn't matter as long as you are consistent. Again, it's not the absolute number, it's the change that matters. It should also be noted that many successful losers like to weigh themselves every day. I'm not one of them, but to each his own.

# ANOTHER TOOL: THE MEETING

So what happens at a Weight Watchers meeting?

Depending on who you are and what you seek, lots of things. I have been to more Weight Watchers meetings than I can count, in locations all over the world, sometimes in languages I do not understand. I have learned a tremendous number of tips, sayings, and other useful bits from both the leaders who run these meetings and the other members who attend them.

This knowledge can vary from reframing the mental process around weight loss to the most basic of eating tips (e.g., dip your fork in a side dish of salad dressing before you spear a lettuce leaf, so you get the flavor with a minimum of calories).

Meetings also help people recognize that a weight problem is not something that they have to shoulder alone. When we recognize that we are all suffering from the same plight, we become stronger by helping one another.

For me, one of the most important aspects of the experience is seeing living, breathing role models who have made big changes in their lives, transforming themselves much more radically than I have. If you spend time with someone who has lost more than 100 pounds, you recognize that there is no challenge you cannot overcome.

# Make Incentives and Goals Count

One of the challenges of dealing with a weight issue is recognizing that you are turning down a muffin now so you can reduce your risk of horrible ailments 20 years from now. Most of us have a pretty predictable response to trade-offs between immediate versus delayed gratification. The threat of type 2 diabetes is real, but is it as real as the muffin in the case at the bakery? We humans are just not wired to eat for tomorrow. We need much more immediate reasons.

## TIP #1: SET SHORT-TERM AND MANAGEABLE GOALS

Imagine starting a weight loss process with a goal of losing 100 pounds, and defining success purely on reaching that milestone. Pretty daunting. Imagine having this goal and then weighing-in, and finding you've lost only half a pound.

Or gained a pound! You're setting yourself up for disappointment.

You're better off if you recognize that incredible health improvements can come with relatively modest weight loss. For example, if an obese person loses 7 to 8 percent of her body weight and sustains that loss, she reduces her risk of getting diabetes by 58 percent! Reaching a healthier weight is not the same thing as auditioning for *People* magazine's sexiest person of the year.

Another good idea is to set goals that are within reach in a month or two. Weight Watchers usually recommends setting a weight loss goal of 5 percent for the first milestone. Achieving a doable goal is a way to put a big win on the scorecard.

# TIP #2: CREATE INCENTIVES THAT WILL MAKE YOUR WEIGHT LOSS MEAN SOMETHING

I have a huge incentive to maintain my weight loss: being the CEO of Weight Watchers. How can I talk the talk with our frontline people, with our members, if I am not obviously walking the walk as well? This has kept me incredibly focused over the past 5 years.

Okay, right, you're not the CEO of Weight Watchers.

People have used lots of techniques to create a sense of urgency to their weight management process. They place bets with friends. They build in rewards for achieving key milestones. They make public commitments to friends and family. They blog and tweet successes and failures.

Bottom line: If you can make yourself feel accountable to someone else, it motivates you to stick to the healthy path.

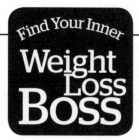

# To change your pant size, cinch it with a tool belt.

## Make sure you've got versatile, easy-to-use instruments.

To make serious lifestyle changes, use tools that help you become more mindful and in control—a Points or calorie tracker, heart rate monitor, scale. The biggest value of tracking for me is that (1) it does not allow me to live in denial of the real impact of my choices, and (2) it makes me much more aware of the little mindless sneaks I so often commit.

## Stop treating the scale as your judge and jury.

Instead, start using it as a motivator. People tend not to freak out when they see a stopwatch before running a lap. They want to know whether they are making progress on their time. The scale is no different.

## Set realistic goals.

When you do set goals for yourself, try to keep the time frame to 1 to 2 months, if not just a couple of weeks. It's much easier to stay focused that way.

## Join up.

Don't be afraid to get support. Seek it out. Have your friends join you.

## Weight Watchers Profile

## "I love myself. I never did before."

Healthy pleasures are satisfying in two ways–feel great now, even better later

**Susan Brilla, 28,** *Liverpool, NY*
**HEIGHT:** 5 feet 9 inches
**WEIGHT BEFORE:** 252
**WEIGHT AFTER:** 160
Reached her goal in 18 months

### MY STRUGGLE

I never paid attention to what I ate—and to top it off, I love beer. By age 24, I was wearing a size 22 and had been diagnosed with endometriosis, a painful uterine condition. To treat it, I had to undergo a 7-month series of shots, causing me to enter menopause pre-maturely. That took a toll not only physically, but also emotionally. I kept think-ing, "I'm 24, and I'm going through all this stuff." I had simply stopped caring for myself and, as a result, had put on 80 pounds in less than 6 months.

### MY WAKE-UP CALL

One day my boyfriend and I were on the way home from his softball team's steak bake. I still felt hungry, so I asked him to stop at KFC. As I was ordering, I actually screamed. It had suddenly occurred to me, "What are you doing? You just ate yourself to death at a steak bake, and now you're in the KFC drive-thru." It didn't help when I saw pictures from a camping trip a few weeks prior. Until then, I had been in denial about how much weight I had gained. But you can't argue with photos.

### MY FOOD

I've learned that depriving myself is the fastest road to failure. So I haven't given up beer entirely. I've just fig-ured out how to fit it in. If I want to have a drink dur-ing the week, I switch to a lighter beer, instead of my favorite craft beers. And I make sure to counteract it with activity, whether it's running, hitting the elliptical, or taking a walk. I now look at beer as a small treat and a way to relax, not to overindulge. This has become the model for my entire diet—I find healthier versions of the things I love. I can easily demolish an entire block of cheese, so I limit myself to light options. If you feel deprived, look at your plate and ask yourself, "What am I not enjoying? What would I enjoy? And how can I make that healthier?"

I've also started using smaller plates—it's a psychological thing. If you have this gigantic plate, you think your portion is tiny, even if it's the 4 ounces of protein you're supposed to have. If you put it on a smaller plate, it looks like more. It's a mind game, but it works.

## MY FITNESS

I started running, but not just for the physical benefit (and the extra beers it lets me drink). When I run by myself, it gives me a chance to clear my head, to refocus on my goals. I started with a half-marathon. Then last year I was able to run my first full marathon!

## MY PAYOFF

My level of confidence has skyrocketed. Before, I never showed my teeth when I smiled—it was just this little smirk. But now. I'm grinning in every picture. I love myself, which I never did before.

# {CHAPTER 8}

# Manage Your Environment

## (Don't Let Your House Become an EPA Superfund Site)

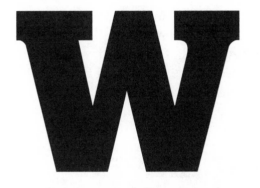HY DO PEOPLE FAIL
TO REACH THEIR
WEIGHT LOSS
**GOALS** or regain
weight they've lost?
One prevailing theory:
They fail to change and
protect their environ-
ment. I'm not talking
about pollution, wet-
lands, or the ozone layer. I'm talking about the food and activity
environment that surrounds us. The contents of our refrigera-
tors and kitchen cabinets. The pathways we travel (or don't) at
lunchtime. The late-night temptations that lurk in our freezers.
All of these can contribute to an energy-dense environment
that takes a toll on our midsections. Alternately, we can rid our
environment of these hazards, so it nourishes and protects us.
But we have to shape our surroundings in a way that will help,
not hurt, us.

We know fairly conclusively that the primary reason our
population has become more obese is that our food and activity environments have changed drastically over the past hundred years, particularly in the last 25. As noted earlier in the
book, the number of calories each of us has available to them
jumped a good (that is, bad) 25 percent over that same quarter
century. If what the scientists call an obesogenic environment is plumping up the populace, then it stands to reason

that living in that environment puts each of us at high risk for unhealthy lifestyle choices.

There are a lot of smart and passionate obesity fighters in the world who recognize the impact that our environment has on us. Many of these folks believe we should aggressively regulate the food industry to banish meaningless calories from the environment. They argue for taxes on soda, fast food, and other obesogens that bring too many of us down.

I don't know if heavy taxes on soda would have the desired outcome, though certainly consuming large quantities of full-sugar soda contributes to obesity. Still, I don't believe that we can or should wait for someone else to try to fix the problem for us. As individuals, we need to take responsibility for our own health, and we'd better do it now.

# What "Environment" Are We Talking About?

It's virtually impossible to make permanent behavior changes if we do not change our environment at the same time. With this in mind, let's define what we really mean by that.

## IN THE BROADER COMMUNITY

Most of us have cheap and easy access to foods with lots of extra sugars, salt, and fats in the public places where we live, dine, and shop. Much of what one can buy these days in the grocery store is unhealthy—overly processed and flavored—at least in excessive quantities, and a glance at most chain restaurant menus reveals too many items clogged with sodium, hidden sugar, and unhealthy fats. That's not how nature intended us to nourish ourselves.

We can't demand that grocers remove half of the items from their shelves any more than we can demand that a restaurant change its menu, but we can influence what the store stocks and the restaurant serves by what we buy. In Chapter 10, I'll equip you with strategies for sidestepping land mines on restaurant menus. When it comes to grocery shopping, you can avoid temptation and grocery cart wrecks by shopping the outer reaches of the store—typically the fruit and vegetable, meat, and dairy sections. That's where the whole foods live, the ones that should constitute most of what you eat. Also: Always shop with a list, and stick to it.

# AT WORK

Many of us spend the majority of our time in our workplaces, whose food environments are typically designed to keep nose to grindstone: cafeterias, vending machines, and catering for meetings. But that convenience can create numerous areas for pitfalls throughout the day. A dish of candies at the end of someone's cubicle or a breakfast catered with a towering platter of pastry delights can bend the will of the best of us. Cafeterias often cater to the lowest common nutritional denominator, so deep fryers and heaps of mac 'n' cheese can reign supreme, next to such obesogen staples as chips and soda.

Work is also the place where we tend to be bored, stressed, anxious, or some exasperating mix of all of the above. Take a bunch of people in those emotional states, mix them with a lot of tasty, comforting treats, and you have a twilight zone of overeating.

# AT HOME

For many of us, this is ground zero for weight gain. We find ourselves prowling around through the kitchen at 9 p.m., looking for a bite here or a handful there. This is where we keep treats for the kids, but we are only too happy to serve them up to ourselves as well. (Just who are we buying them for, really?) At least at work, we have the benefit of a fairly busy pace, and we also might be reluctant to kick off a serious binge with our colleagues watching our every move. At home, we're shielded from prying eyes, which can give free rein to mindless and private eating. The good news about our home environment is that we can—we *should*—control every bit of food that comes into it.

# Why Our Environment Is Such a Big Deal

Throughout this section, you will hear me frequently cite a food psychology genius by the name of Brian Wansink, who has served up a vast buffet of tasty research at Cornell University. His life's work is looking into the ways that people interact with food, and he concocts lots of ingenious ways to do that.

One specific finding by Dr. Wansink's research team has heavily influenced the way I think about our obesogenic environment. In one study, they found that their test subjects made around 220 food decisions each day; yet these same test subjects estimated that they make just 15 food and beverage decisions per day.

How can people make 205 separate decisions each day and not realize it? The simple answer is: Most of these decisions are split-second considerations that people are only vaguely, if at all, aware of.

Take the following scenario: I'm sitting in a meeting, which has been catered with trays of pastries and various other breakfast foods. Every time I look at the food display, I'm making a decision not to get up and grab another cheese Danish. I might easily do that 20 to 25 times over a 2-hour period—more often, if somebody starts lingering over his PowerPoint presentation. When food is in front of us, we react to it. It's part of our animal nature, going back to the days when we were chasing mastodons with our pointy sticks.

So, if we are making 200-plus weight-related decisions each day, can we be trusted to make good ones? Possibly not, according to some recent research from Jonathan Levav of Stanford and Shai Danziger of Ben-Gurion University. Their study looked at the ability of courtroom judges to make good decisions without breaks, which led them to conclude that having to make too many decisions can lead to a state of decision fatigue. After a while, our brain begins to tire of having to make choice after choice, deliver verdict after verdict. If we are making too many, our brains start looking for short-cuts, which lead us to make impulsive choices.

In this context, Dr. Wansink's research is all the more cause for alarm. If we were locked in a room filled with all of the foods we love, we would almost certainly break down and start eating them. This may seem like an unlikely scenario, but on some level this is what's happening to each of us all day, every day. We no longer kill what we eat; it's served up to us on an endless conveyor belt during our waking hours.

# Pity Our Poor Brains

We've all experienced the sensation of being slightly out of control when food is right in front of us. Arguably, part of our desire to eat is just habit, but is it also possible that there is a physiological process in play?

A couple of years ago, I attended the International Congress on Obesity in Stockholm, Sweden. That's where I learned about some fascinating research on what our brains look like when we're hungry. Functional magnetic resonance imaging (fMRI) shows neural activity as it is actually happening, as cool colors light up the gray matter to show our food lust.

Researchers use this technology to explore which parts of the brain are activated by different stimuli. Some researchers now theorize that there are two pathways that show how brain activity processes hunger.

**The homeostatic system:** This is basically the control mechanism our bodies use to manage our energy balance. The brain triggers a release of hormones to either stimulate (ghrelin) or suppress (leptin) hunger, depending on how much we've eaten. This system was designed to help us figure out when we need food or not, though it doesn't necessarily guide people to their swimsuit-fantasy selves.

This finely tuned system regulates how our body maintains energy balance. When we try to lose weight, we reduce energy intake and our bodies react to the changes. Next step: We start feeling hungry.

**The hedonic system:** This appetite driver guides people to consume "highly palatable" foods by releasing dopamine, the pleasure-reward hormone. Basically, when you see chocolate cake, your brain goes into reward-seeking mode. And you eat. Or you really want to eat. Badly. This system is our desire for pleasure and reward. It operates in addition to the homeostatic system.

Recent research demonstrates that the hedonic system goes into overdrive for people who struggle with their weight (like me). Our brains light up like a Christmas tree when we see something yummy. Apparently, the naturally thin do not have this neural fireworks display to nearly the same degree.

Fortunately, someone who has lost weight and kept it off has "activated" a separate brain structure (the dorsal lateral prefrontal cortex, in case you were wondering) that lights up when it detects something yummy. This is the part that helps us rein in our impulsive behaviors. A friend asked me if such a brain structure could be implanted or purchased. You can't buy one on Amazon yet, but you may be able to develop it, like new muscle, through practice and training.

So what's my personal take on all of the above?

I totally relate to these theories. My brain gets fuzzy when I see my favorite trigger foods. I cannot look at a muffin without my heart's skipping a beat and a weird buzzing sensation in my head. At the same time, I am now pretty adept at not eating said muffin as long as it's not right in front of me. Over the years, I've built up my self-restraint muscles to the point where I can hold back. But I still need to avoid being around those foods that make my brain-heart go pitter-pat.

I find it interesting to see how my various impulses are correlated to neuroscience. Still, I find it all kind of obvious: We need to find ways to battle our cravings. None of that is brain surgery. At least I hope not.

# Is Food Lust Related to the Other Kind?

We all know about public people who have made disastrous decisions in their private lives. What were they thinking when they tweeted that photo or unseemly proposal? What made them act so impulsively?

Does that kind of self-destructive behavior happen when we are in a state of frenzied food lust?

Who best to answer this question? Why, an economist of course! Behavioral economists spend their time figuring out how human beings make decisions. Those 200-plus food-related choices Brian Wansink wrote about? Behavioral economists study how we make them. They offer interesting perspectives on how people choose among foods on grocery store shelves, why they order what they do at restaurants, and how they decide whether or not to lace up their running shoes on a Saturday afternoon.

*Nudge: Improving Decisions about Health, Wealth, and Happiness* is an interesting book that delves into these topics at some length. The basic tenet of the authors—Richard Thaler, an economics professor at the University of Chicago, and Cass Sunstein, law professor at Harvard—is that by better understanding our decision-making processes, we can help nudge ourselves and others toward better choices. We at Weight Watchers are prime nudgers, so how could I not see these guys as kindred spirits?

The authors delve into the automatic versus reflective systems of the mind: One is instinctive and impulsive, and the other is planning oriented and analytic. We need both to navigate our incredibly complicated day-to-day world. I'm glad that I don't have to weigh the pros and cons of breathing or laughing at a joke. At the same time, if I was instinctive 100 percent of the time, I would probably be running naked through the streets of Manhattan right now.

When it comes to food, it's pretty easy for me to see my automatic system in action. It is the part of my brain that leads to mindless eating. In one particularly fascinating part of the book, Thaler and Sunstein draw distinctions between the mind's cold states (i.e., food is not in front of us) and hot states (we have a bowl of nuts in our lap). As they delicately put it: "For most of us, self-control issues arise because we underestimate the effect of arousal." They continue, "When in a cold state, we do not appreciate how much our desires and our behavior will be altered when we are 'under the influence' of arousal."

Say what?

My interpretation: When we fall under a food spell, we can fall to pieces. As always, I'm happy to oblige with my own miserable example.

I was flying back from Brussels to New York right after I read *Nudge*. I told myself the following things before I boarded the plane: no wine or nuts, certainly no cheese plates, only low-fat dishes. I nearly made it. I didn't graze in the airport lounge. I said "No thanks" to the preflight cocktails, opting for a Diet Coke instead. Then something snapped inside me. When the flight attendant put a small bowl of nuts in front of me, I totally succumbed to my "arousal state." I was "hot" and ate everything else they gave me before falling asleep (or was it hibernation?).

When I awoke, the hot state was past, replaced by memory and shame. So I was able to turn down the snack offered at the end of the flight. But I had already lost it big-time.

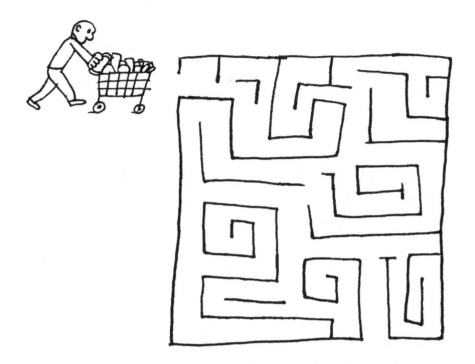

What's the moral of all of this? I can't try to beat my own brain. If I test myself too much, I'm going to fail eventually and maybe catastrophically. But that is the value of controlling my environment: I can't get aroused by what I don't have in front of me. The best way to avoid a "hot state" is to surround oneself with cool, icy, inedible objects.

Business class on an airplane is arousal central for me. I'm strapped to a chair for 8 hours and surrounded by people succumbing to their own hot states. I travel a lot, but thankfully the total number of airplane meals and temptations are manageable. It makes more sense for me to prioritize my efforts when I'm on solid ground, to fix environments I can control.

So after my trip to Brussels, the first thing I did was stock the house with fruit and healthy snacks. I stayed "cold" for the next few days and felt much better for it.

My golden rule in weight loss and maintenance (for myself, anyway) is to accept the limitations of my own will-power. Probably because of my own automatic systems and hot states, I cannot rely on it to always help me slam on the brakes. Planning and environmental control are the keys to my long-term success.

That, and apparently taking more cold showers.

# Fastest Eater in 7 States:
# My Life of Food Rush

When food is put in front of me, I notice the following changes in my physiology: My pulse quickens, my eyes lock into tunnel vision, I'm coated with a thin film of perspiration, my sense of smell heightens, and I begin salivating like a dog in the presence of a nice juicy squirrel. It must be disturbing for my wife and family to observe me in this state, when husband/daddy takes on the appearance of a high-RPM windmill-like device, wielding spoons/forks at the end of each fan blade to rapidly deposit food in a bottomless mouthlike pit.

I call this bodily frenzy of mine Food Rush. Obesity researchers refer to it as food anticipation. It's a disastrous way to approach a plate of food. My mind has no time to determine if I'm still hungry as I scrape down to the shiny finish on the plate. Food Rush is certainly one of the factors that led to my charter membership in the Clean Plate Club.

Recently, I was watching my dog, Gabby, eat her breakfast, and it occurred to me that Food Rush is a behavior common to many a large dog. I used a stopwatch to see how long it took Gabby to blow through her food. The count: precisely 56 seconds to down a large bowl of chow.

I'm not much different.

I typically eat as fast as humanly possible, preferably without taking a breath. I have to consciously decide to set the fork down after a bite. But if I force myself to be aware of how fast I'm eating, I can successfully slow down. My primary point in sharing this man-dog link is to demonstrate that we're not all Gabbys. We know that our brains can get us in trouble, but we can also ask them to help us behave.

# Visual Distortion and Willpower
## (Not a Fair Fight)

In the world of weight management, the word I despise the most is willpower. It bothers me that there is a presumption that if we were just "better" people, there would not be an obesity issue in this country. Dealing with a weight issue does require attention and elbow grease, but our failings are not owing to a lack of character.

This brings me back to Brian Wansink and the clever experiments that he and his colleagues have undertaken to understand how we behave around food. Wansink possesses a weird combination of intelligence, statistical rigor, and a slightly diabolical sense of humor.

Those are good qualities in a researcher and in an author, and they're fully on display in his book *Mindless Eating: Why We Eat More Than We Think*. (No, he didn't dedicate it to me, though he could have.) His main theory is that we tend to overestimate our ability to resist temptations in our environment. His advice: Don't try to summon mythical heaps of willpower, but rather adapt your environment to encourage healthier choices.

One of Dr. Wansink's cornerstone observations is that very few people stop eating because they are full. Rather, they drop the fork when they receive certain external cues. In one particularly twisted experiment, he asked a bunch of test subjects to eat soup until they were full. All of us members of the Clean Plate Club use the existence of an empty plate as a signal that we must be full. But he and his coconspirators rigged some 18-ounce soup bowls so that they refilled automatically. Unbeknownst to his test subjects, they either sat down in front of a normal bowl or bellied up to a bottomless one.

Here were the results.

- **People in the normal bowl group (if 18 ounces can be considered normal) ate an average of 9 ounces of soup.** When asked to estimate how many calories they thought they consumed, they guessed 123. It turns out they actually ate 153 calories. In other words, they underestimated by 24 percent—a cautionary tale for us all!

- **People in the bottomless bowl group ate an average of 15 ounces (!), or 67 percent more than the normal bowl group.** Apparently a few ate over a quart. When asked how many calories they guessed they had eaten, they came up with an average of 127—about the same as the normal-bowl group. In fact, they had eaten an average of 268 calories, underestimating by 111 percent how much they had eaten.

We can thank Dr. Wansink for informing us not to lay in a supply of bowls that magically refill. But his other assist comes from reinforcing the lesson that human beings are terrible at guesstimating calories. We also haven't a clue about when to stop eating, especially if our dishware doesn't provide it for us. Most research indicates that it takes the stomach about 20 minutes to inform the brain that it's had enough food. I don't think I've ever taken 20 minutes to blast through a plate of food in my entire life.

Those bottomless bowls remind us, as well, why keeping track of what we eat is so important. Countless studies support Dr. Wansink's finding that people have a strong tendency to underestimate how much they eat. Their guesses come up short by 25 to 30 percent most of the time. That is more than enough of an error to result in consistent weight gain, and it can explain why many of us have trouble losing weight or keeping it off. Even when we track, we have a tendency to underestimate portion size or "forget" to track bites/licks/tastes. Still, the act of tracking has been demonstrated again and again to give trackers a huge advantage in attaining their goals.

I'll give you an example of how Dr. Wansink's theories play out in my daily life. Our neighbors invited us over for a barbecue. They set out a full spread of food, particularly on the chips and guacamole side of the table. I have no earthly idea how much I ate, other than the fact that it was a heck of a lot more than I could ever hope to guess at.

What would have been a better strategy? Easy (in theory— not necessarily practice). Rather than pick off the finger food trays, I should have plated everything I planned to eat. I could have easily lingered and nibbled off the plate, but I would have had a visual cue when I was getting to the end. Another nice benefit of preplating snacks is that it forces me through a series of steps that are slightly more involved and deliberate, unlike my too-frequent practice of opening a bag, shoving my head inside of it, and then breathing deeply.

# Of Little Plates and Full Tummies

Earlier in the book, I described the food plate icon that the Departments of Agriculture and HHS released to reinforce the new *Dietary Guidelines for Americans* (see page 85). Half of the plate is reserved for fruits and vegetables, and the rest holds whole grains and lean proteins. There's also a serving of low-fat dairy on the side, to whet the whistle with more protein and calcium. I like the new icon a lot and see it as a huge improvement over the old food pyramid, which we can all agree was a confusing failure.

Why is the plate better? Two reasons:

- **I like what it says.** The cutting-edge advice in food choices is pretty simple and common sense: Eat real foods that have real nutrition. This is what the PointsPlus System is all about, and it reflects the way I eat (or at least aspire to) these days.

- **I like how it says it.** I have never served my food on a pyramid. But I relate to the plate. Visualizing the divisions between fruits and vegetables, whole grains, and protein, makes a lot of sense to me. Nothing like a simple message to penetrate the density of my skull.

Still, there is another distinction that doesn't really find its way onto the new plate icon: portion control. How big a plate are we talking about? One of Dr. Wansink's bottomless bowls? A platter?

There was an amusing study published recently that looked at artistic renderings of the Last Supper over the past 1,000 years. Visual analysis compared the size of plates and loaves of bread to the size of heads in the paintings, so researchers were able to measure how artistic interpretations of serving sizes had changed. Over the past millennium, those artistic plate sizes have increased an average of 66 percent, with the biggest gains coming around the year 1500. I guess no one can blame Coke and Pepsi for that one.

Over the course of the 1990s, average plate sizes have grown from 10 inches to 12 inches, an increase of 20 percent. Does this matter? According to Dr. Wansink, it matters quite a bit.

Time for another round of human experimentation in the Cornell labs.

• **EXPERIMENT #1:** At an ice-cream social (the opposite of a Weight Watchers meeting), the researchers gave their test subjects either 17-ounce bowls or 34-ounce bowls. Those who were given the larger bowls served themselves 31 percent more ice cream. When given a larger scoop to go with their great big bowl, they dished out 57 percent more ice cream.

• **EXPERIMENT #2:** Test subjects served a medium-size hamburger on a smaller plate (a saucer) estimated their burger to have 18 percent more calories than when it was served on a regulation-size plate.

Clearly, our eyes deceive us when we try to judge serving sizes and calorie counts. Maybe this is why fancy restaurants are often accused of skimping on food: They put normal portions on huge plates.

I have two observations.

First, appetizers can be pleasant surprises. I was recently invited to speak to a bunch of Wall Street types about Weight Watchers. I knew they'd be grilling me for the main course, so I didn't bother ordering an entrée. Instead, I asked for an appetizer serving of tuna tartare. When it arrived, it looked kind of impressive on its smaller dish. So I wolfed it down and then kept my mouth busy with my talk for the rest of lunch. I ended up feeling pretty satisfied afterward and wasn't hungry again until dinner. Moral of the story? It's either: A small plate makes for a satisfying meal (no matter how much is on it), or I should just talk more and eat less.

Second, I am not wired to leave food on a plate. My choice is either to fight this urge or simply to use a smaller plate. Given the plate inflation of the last hundred years, if you pick up salad plates now, they'll be about the size of dinner plates 20 years ago. Less surface area on the plate will mean less surface area on your body.

# Suffer from Overgrazing?
## Fence Off Your Kitchen!

Sometimes I have to laugh at myself and my bizarre methods for keeping a grip on eating reality.

Despite all of my progress in cleaning up my act, I still have my danger zones. One of my biggest is a special cabinet in our kitchen that houses various baking supplies and a few snacks. This is where I go when I'm just home from work (i.e., before dinner) or when I'm wandering the kitchen on the weekends.

So what's the draw in this irresistible cabinet? Recently it's been full of nuts, chocolate chips, and a very large bag of M&M's—all intended for baking, not for stuffing David. My wife is an active and proficient chef, presiding over the fine dining at Chez Kirchhoff. Recently, my two girls have joined her staff, and my 11-year-old loves to bake cookies. But not as much as I love pilfering her ingredients.

That large bag of candy was intended to be used for cookies for a school bake sale. But there was a change of plans, and the M&M's went untouched. Fortunately for me, they were sealed; I do not steal from sealed bags of ingredients. My preferred method is to sneak imperceptible quantities of chocolate chips and nuts in delta force–worthy stealth attacks. However, if the bag stays closed or tightly sealed, I leave it be. This all works very well until the bag is opened, which it finally was. Sure enough I started grabbing small handfuls of M&M's every 3 or 4 days. Not terrible, but it's also the kind of grazing habit I'm trying to quit.

What could I do given that the bag of M&M's was fairly giant in size? In a moment of utter brilliance, I put a bag of flour on top of it as a deterrent. Seriously, I did this, and I haven't had an M&M since. Apparently, seeing the bag has been an adequate reminder to me that I should not sneak.

What about almonds? They're healthy, right? Well, they are most definitely healthy, but they are also disturbingly dense with energy. I started getting the prepackaged Trader Joe's almonds, thinking that this could help me avoid my eat-'em-by-the-handful habit. However, a small premade bag is still enough to hold 38 of the little buggers, which racks up a big caloric hit. Not terrible if this is the only thing I'm eating beyond dinner, but not really the stuff intended for a mindless bite before dinner.

I guess it takes all kinds of efforts to control one's private obesogenic microclimate. I can track with the best of them in the morning and afternoon, but after three years on maintenance, I still have a hard time keeping the thread in the evening. Particularly those post–6 p.m. bites, licks, and tastes. And then there's the no-man's-land of the weekend. Forcing myself to at least acknowledge the impact of these danger zones could help keep me out of the M&M's bag.

As I considered the effect of those indulgences, it was a quick step over to the liquor cabinet to see what damage I was doing there. Quite some time ago, I developed a fondness for an evening glass of bourbon on the rocks. I can nurse one for well over an hour, and it just seems so civilized and restrained. Should be no problem, right? Wrong. It seems that one of those short glasses, with ice, is still enough to hold ½ cup (4 ounces) of bourbon. What's the price? About 276 bloody calories. Crud. It makes the 5-ounce pour of wine at half the calorie cost seem like a bargain.

The whole exercise was a little sad, exposing my own sloppy tendencies, but I suppose that knowledge is power. It gives me an extra reason to look into alternative strategies for both snacks and drinks. Sneaking around is just not worth the hit I'm taking, right in the gut.

# Managing Your Environment

Solve your environmental problem, and you have a real shot at setting yourself up for success. Develop a line of attack following the plan below.

Know your weaknesses. My wife always laughs at the way I grow visibly agitated if I see an unopened box of cookies. But she's the same way with a jar of nuts. Each of us has weaknesses that cause our brains to go fuzzy. Know what they are and you can find a solution that defuses the issue.

Barricade the gates and watch the sight lines. Recognize which foods will beat you nine fights out of 10. Don't tempt yourself. Create a physical condition or visual cue that will remind you not to reach for them. My personal favorite is to keep these foods out of sight. I have been known to ask my family to keep ice-cream containers in the downstairs freezer so I don't see them. Okay, yes, this makes me look like a child with zero impulse control, but I really don't want to battle my brain over it. Out of sight, out of mouth.

Make the better alternatives easily accessible. Once the dangerous foods are inconveniently located, I set the healthy ones right at hand. I make sure that there is an ample supply of grapes or strawberries within sight and grasp, if I need a fix. I also substitute Greek yogurt mixed with frozen berries for ice-cream bars. Finally, if I really need to dip, then I will make sure I've got carrot and celery sticks along with a low-calorie bean dip. It actually tastes great.

If you create an environment in your home that nudges you to make better decisions, you will find yourself making those decisions. If you do not, you will find yourself endlessly fighting your urges, and many times you will lose.

In this casino, you can stack the deck in your favor. Why wouldn't you do that?

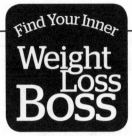

## Set yourself up for success by slaying the dragons all around you.

### Don't fight it.
Respect the environment. If we put ourselves into tempting situations—confronting our dragons—every 5 minutes, we will eventually fold. The key is to reengineer your personal environment so you don't *have* to battle temptation.

### Predict your "hot states."
Our brains can get us into trouble, but they can also help us behave. If you know what kinds of foods arouse you, you can better manage your environment and surround yourself with things that leave you cold. If a box of cookies causes you to crumble, put them someplace you don't see them every time you open the cabinet door.

### Be mindful, and use visual tricks.
Few people stop eating because they're full. Your eyes *are* bigger than your stomach. If I force myself to be aware of how fast I'm eating, I can successfully slow down and know when I'm feeling sated. To control portion size, use a smaller plate.

### Make the better options easily accessible.
Keep a supply of healthier foods at hand—fresh and frozen fruit, cut vegetables, Greek yogurt, low-calorie bean dip—for when a craving hits and so deprivation doesn't set in.

## Weight Watchers Profile

## "I'm setting goals... and surprising myself."

Sometimes one step at a time turns into one marathon at a time

**Melanie Kann, 33,** *Queens, NY*
**HEIGHT:** 5 feet 5 inches
**WEIGHT BEFORE:** 167
**WEIGHT AFTER:** 128
Reached her goal in 6 months

### MY STRUGGLE

It's funny because I never actually gained weight. I kind of always was the way I was. When I was little, I was taller than all the other kids in the grade. I was just bigger than them, thus my nickname "Thunder Thighs." I never thought of myself as an overweight person until I went shopping with my friends when I was a little older. My jeans were a double-digit size, while theirs were a single digit. I realized there was a big difference.

### MY WAKE-UP CALL

I'm an actress. Before my weight loss, I was starring in a four-person Frank Sinatra revue, and none of the costumes would fit me. They pulled out all of these things that either were for teeny tiny skinny people or for a size 20. I was like "Do you really see me as that large of a person? You really think I would fit into that giant costume?" And the woman said, "Well, we can just cinch the waist." I went to the director crying. And I was like "I can't, I'm supposed to be pretty." The costumer ended up sewing me a custom dress. Utter embarrassment.

### MY FOOD

You hear stories about people who eat for emotional reasons. That was never me. I just had no idea that the foods I was eating were bad for me. I didn't know that having a bagel with cream cheese for breakfast, a tomato mozzarella basil sandwich with chicken and a cookie for lunch, and four big sushi rolls for dinner was too much. For me, it was really about accountability and education.

**MY FITNESS**
I hate the gym, so I used to play tricks to make myself go. My favorite: locking my keys and gym bag in the locker at the New York Sports Club on my way to work. This forced me to go to the gym on my way home. But I was miserable. So I started walking. Walking became jogging, and at a friend's suggestion,

I signed up for my first race. I found something I love, and that helped me push myself. Even now, eight marathons later, I'm still pushing myself. I'm still setting goals to keep me motivated. I keep surprising myself.

**MY PAYOFF**
Before my weight loss, I always felt like I was being miscast as an actor—I'd play crazy old ladies, nuns, people who didn't have to wear tight clothes. I thought people weren't seeing me. Now I'm more comfortable onstage, which means I can embrace my roles and have fun with them, no matter what they are!

# {CHAPTER 9}

# Maintenance:
## How to Dance Down the Long Road Ahead

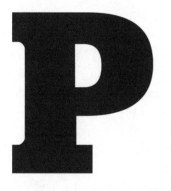**ARDON ME** while I brag a little bit. As I write this passage, I have been a Lifetime Member of Weight Watchers for 33 months. I achieved that hard-fought distinction on March 17, 2009. I consider the shrinking of me one of the biggest accomplishments of my life.

So what exactly am I bragging about?

Lifetime Membership is a special designation that Weight Watchers uses to recognize people who have reached a healthy weight—generally defined as a BMI of 25 or below—and stay there for at least 6 weeks. Once they become a Lifetime Member, they are recognized for their achievement and are entitled to attend Weight Watchers meetings for free, as long as they stay within 2 pounds of their goal weight and weigh in at least once a month.

I have met Lifetime Members who have been at their goal weight for more than 25 years. I have even met a few Lifetime Members who can trace their experience all the way back to our founder, Jean Nidetch. I have met other Lifetime Members who lost their way, regained their weight, and had to start over with the program to lose it again.

What all of them will tell you, me included, is that maintenance is challenging. Yet it's a manageable challenge, especially because there are so many rewards that come with meeting it.

One of the difficult truths all of us have to recognize is that if you have had a problem with weight, in some sense you will always have a problem with weight. It never really goes away. While we can rise to the challenge and manage our weight, it will always require a certain amount of effort and diligence. In this context, it might be best to think of a weight problem as a sort of chronic condition.

My problem, maybe yours too, is that for all of my efforts to stick with healthier habits, I continue to face the same conditions that led me to gain weight in the first place. The food environment that led to rising obesity is still present. This means that all of the temptation to which we have previously succumbed (and sometimes still do) is still there. It seems unlikely that our food environment will ever return to the conditions circa 1950—small plates, reasonable portions, and scarce fast food. They are gone forever.

Further, according to studies on behavior change, there is a sizable risk of recidivism. Backsliding is a probability, if not a certainty. For one thing, turning to food for emotional reasons is deeply programmed and very hard to overcome. Combine our changeable emotions with a food environment built to stuff us to the gills, and the road forward begins to look like a traffic circle, looping us back past the same hazards over and over.

So, for a reality check, anyone going through a weight loss process can expect the following to occur:

- You will have bad days and possibly bad weeks.
- You have a good chance of regaining weight you lost.
- You will become discouraged.

Now the good news. If you accept that all of the above will happen, you have a great shot at rising above these challenges and emerging even stronger. You can absolutely maintain weight loss over time if you recognize that this process requires steady attention to a few important details.

# Basic Truths about Weight Maintenance

There is a whole branch of research that seems to devote itself to the sole purpose of discouraging us from even trying to lose weight. Depressingly, it suggests that those of us who drop a few pounds are somehow doomed to regain them. As if it's natural law that we give up, give in, and accept our unhealthy fate.

I don't live my life that way, and I don't want anybody assuming that of you, either.

Being a positive guy, I focus on an equal and opposite body of research that suggests that people can sustainably maintain weight loss. For example, a study of Weight Watchers Lifetime Members showed that 47 percent had maintained at least a 10 percent weight loss after 2 years. More comprehensively, there is a wonderful source of research on this topic from the aforementioned National Weight Control Registry.

This long-term research study tracks 10,000 people whom I consider among my personal heroes: They've lost weight, are keeping it off, and are sharing the details with the rest of us who need help. Here are some characteristics shared by that mob of successful losers.

- Eighty percent of the subjects in the registry are women and 20 percent are men. (Come on, guys, let's show some effort here.)

- The average woman in the study is 45 years old and weighs 145 pounds, while the average man is 49 years old and weighs 190 pounds.

- Registry members have each lost an average of 66 pounds and kept the weight off for 5.5 years.

- At the extremes, they lost between 30 and 300 pounds.

- The duration of their successful weight loss has ranged from 1 year to 66 years!

- Some dropped the weight rapidly, others lost it very slowly—over as many as 14 years.

## Other factors they have in common . . .

- 45 percent lost the weight on their own, and the other 55 percent lost weight with the help of some type of program.

- 98 percent report that they modified their food intake in some way to lose weight.

- 94 percent increased their physical activity, most commonly by walking.

There is wide variety in how these members keep the weight off. Most report sticking to a low-calorie, low-fat diet and doing high levels of physical activity.

- 78 percent eat breakfast every day.

- 75 percent weigh themselves at least once a week.

- 62 percent watch less than 10 hours of TV per week.

- 90 percent exercise, on average, about 1 hour per day.

Cold statistical analysis, maybe. But they represent some beautiful turnarounds in very real lives, and they point to paths we can all follow to achieve results that last a lifetime.

# Pick a Plan You Can Live With

Research on these 10,000 role models has shown that their food habits, whatever they were, remained the same in maintenance—often for years—as they were when losing weight. In other words, the kinds of foods that I ate during my weight loss process are exactly the kinds of foods I need to eat now that I'm maintaining my weight. It's the cardinal rule to beat recidivism: Whatever you are doing to lose weight must be what you are willing to do forever. So make it good.

This finding also explains the peril of "dieting." If a diet is a siege we undertake to lose weight as fast as possible, what happens once we reach our goal? Most likely, we revert to our prior habits and watch in horror and amazement as the weight returns, sure as high tide follows low. That's why I don't like to rely on prepackaged meals. Unless I'm willing to sign up for a lifetime delivery plan, it doesn't make sense for me to count on them to lose weight. When the packages stop arriving, I'll take a special delivery right at the waistline. It's an entirely different proposition to use prepackaged meals as a form of periodic convenience, in which case they can be a great help to sustaining a healthier lifestyle.

The fact is, our bodies just can't deal with a state of deprivation. We can tell ourselves that it is okay to be hungry while we are losing weight. We can live with any amount of discomfort for a short time. But if we are still feeling deprived and constantly hungry on maintenance, we will quit the plan to stop the pain.

I attribute much of my success to foods that helped me maintain energy balance but were also satisfying. I filled out my food roster with fruit, oatmeal, and other foods that filled me up but not out—you can find a list in Chapter 4—and they remain my go-to foods to this very day.

## FEEDBACK IS CRITICAL

Three-quarters of the Weight Loss Registry's 10,000 suc-cessful losers weighed themselves at least once a week, sometimes every day. They used that spinning dial as a way of facing the truth about their food intake and energy out-put. Most of these subjects would then set a mental marker denoting how much above their goal weight was acceptable. Once they passed this level, they would immediately return to weight loss mode. For most of them, their tolerance was a 5-to-7-pound gain.

# It's about Food and Exercise

Ten thousand people cannot be entirely wrong. So I tend to perk up when I hear that 94 percent increased their physical activity to lose weight and an astounding 90 percent exer-cise an hour per day. Are they all superhumans with steely personal discipline and endless exercise time? This seems unlikely; they would never have tipped the scales in the first place if they were exercise gods. Rather, the people in this panel were able to make exercise a reality because:

**1.** They made it a priority and carved out time in their busy schedules.

**2.** They built a routine around it so that it became automatic (i.e., a habit).

I may be projecting a bit here. I'm busy, but I carve out time. And I truly need a routine to prevent my lazy self from calling off the gym session. Exercise isn't the silver bullet, as previously discussed, but it does give me some flexibility to periodically stray from my food plan. Super Bowl Sunday, for instance. Plenty of time for a workout before the late-day kickoff—and all of the food that follows.

However, if I simply worked out a lot and ate indiscriminately, I would surely regain my weight. It's far easier to shed calories by not eating certain foods than it is to burn off an indiscretion at the gym. But the two can neatly reinforce each other.

Need more incentive? Consider that building muscle can help you burn more calories at rest (i.e., boost your metabolism) and that cardiovascular exercise burns calories above and beyond. If you are worried about your metabolism slowing after weight loss, this is a great way to counteract it.

Therefore, to really succeed in this endeavor, we need to live a life where we eat smart and stay active and vibrant. Two sides, same coin. Heads you win, tails you win bigger.

Now that I put it that way, it seems pretty straightforward, right?

# Staying Focused

I sometimes think about healthy eating the same way I think about safe driving. (Not that I'm a safe driver. I'll work on that for the next book.) If we stop looking in the rearview mirror, ignore our blind spot, and blow off the speed limit, we can fully expect loud crunching noises coming from the back rear quarter panel. With driving, however, the fear of a horrible death helps keep our eyes on the road. How can we create a similar sense of urgency when it comes to weight? What's the wreck we're avoiding?

Two of my favorite focal points are goal setting and accountability.

## KEEP SETTING GOALS

When you are losing weight, you are at war. It's easier to stay focused. When you are on maintenance, you are living in peacetime. This can be challenging for an old weight loss soldier like myself.

So I invent battles as needed. The doctor's visit. The vacation in some warm place where I'll be seen half naked. The seasonal change of clothes; will they still fit me? Setting short-term goals with implied rewards—I just love it when the doctor congratulates me on my glucose uptake, for instance—is a useful tool for giving maintenance a level of urgency.

## BE ACCOUNTABLE

For all of my statements that we're in this together, that we share common temptations and strengths, there is one thing I have that you don't: a job that would make it really, really

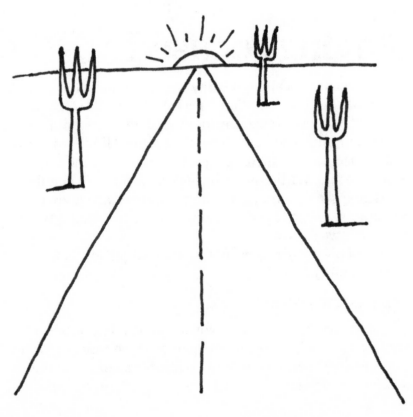

embarrassing if I went on a bender and added 25 pounds.
I really have no choice but to keep the weight off if I want to
keep my job on.

In a significant way, writing my blog—and now a book—
further ups the ante. I'm now publicly blathering to an audience about my healthy lifestyle. In truth, the people who write
in the blog comments section are a pretty kind bunch, but
I still don't want to let them (or you) down. I really need to
keep it together.

Of course, not everybody can be the CEO of Weight Watchers. At least, not all at once. So you could reasonably ask:
Shouldn't the rewards of a healthier lifestyle (and a thinner
profile) be enough to keep me (or anyone else) on program?
Shouldn't I, of all people, be able to do this solely for the benefits of the pursuit itself?

My answer: I can use all the help I can get. We all can.

Life has a way of propelling us into perilous situations.
Throw in a tough economy, a demanding job, and a busy
nuclear family, and circumstances can get really distracting.
The next thing you know, my hand could be sneaking into
the M&M's bag, unobserved.

Short of taking my job, what can you do? Join message
boards, write your own blog, tweet your gains and losses.
I have met some who have made public proclamations to their
families and others who have engaged in weight loss wager-
ing, as I have. For more than a million people each week, the
Weight Watchers meeting (including the all-important weigh-
in) is the most important mechanism for staying accountable
and getting support and encouragement.

My point: We both need to seek support from others and
to have others hold us accountable.

# BE COMPETITIVE

One Sunday morning, I won the fight against daylight sav-
ings time and made my 8:30 a.m. Spinning class. I ended
up working my tail off and did everything I could to throw

myself into cardiac arrest. No loafing on the handlebar, as my Spin teacher has occasionally accused me of doing. So what was the difference? Throughout the class, I kept looking around to see who was working harder. Who was sweating more? When my awesome, cruel teacher asked everyone to bump up their resistance, who was actually doing it? Who was working harder than I was?

A good Spin class has more than its share of mutant cyborgs who seem to have no regard for their own pain and suffering. When they push themselves, I push myself. When they crank the resistance so high that they can barely turn their knobs, I try to join them there in Painland.

I fully embrace the concept of group support—there is nothing I wouldn't do to help a fellow member in a meeting. But personally, I need a little blood sport with my weight loss/maintenance. I need to compete. (I can even beat you at being lazy—don't test me!) When it's me versus the next guy, I want to work harder; I push myself more, stay engaged, stay focused.

My love of competition does not mean I want to lose more weight than everyone else. It's just that I can't stand the idea of people being better at it than me. And because I know lots of people who are better at it, their mere existence helps keep me in the game.

# Thinking about the Real Rewards

For me, one of the hardest parts of weight maintenance has been to fully accept that my new life is my only life. It has been critical for me to see healthy and nutritionally dense foods as the only right foods. Through TV commercials for outstanding desserts and repeated choruses of "I'm lovin' it," we've been brainwashed to think of unhealthy foods as "rewards" and nutritious foods as "work." Because we're going up against that kind of pudge propaganda, it's no wonder that we sometimes lose our grip on healthy habits. I try to remember the following as a useful mental exercise to help me refocus my wayward brain.

Eating healthfully—for good—can seem overwhelming if you think about it too much. Must I count every calorie for the rest of my life? Will I always have to wake up at the crack of dawn to squeeze in a workout? Are breakfast burritos so wrong? I've been good. Don't I deserve my beloved 3,000-calorie megadeath cheeseburger and fries combo? I find I'm better able to handle this so-called workload when I consider the real rewards that await me.

- I feel better physically and mentally when I eat right and don't stuff myself.

- I feel better mentally when I don't pilfer treats in the middle of the night.

- I feel better physically and mentally when I am getting regular exercise. I can't remember a single workout that made me feel worse afterward.

- I am improving my odds to live a longer, less sickly life, and to have many more productive, fun years with my family.

- Truthfully, I look better as a fit guy than as my heavier self. There, I said it. I'm so vain, I probably think this book is about me. But vanity is motivating. You know it. I know it.

My new life, in action: I went to dinner the other night with a big crew of friends. They pretty much all ordered whatever they felt like eating, and I had a nice piece of cod. Should I have thrown in the towel and succumbed to a massive piece of fatty red meat, basted in blue cheese sauce?

I might have, except I actually wanted the cod.

- My fish was terrifically tasty and satisfying. It was a million miles from a hardship.

• I ate plenty. I'm not physically hungry much anymore, as I've found lots of ways to accomplish bulk eating without lots of calories.

• Exercise is no longer a hardship. It's hard to push yourself while you are in the act, but the aftereffect is always worth it.

• My nostalgia for my megadeath days is purely in my head; if I could travel back there, I wouldn't.

# Letting Go Occasionally

Weight Watchers has done an enormous amount of research to understand why someone quits a weight loss or weight maintenance effort. My old boss used to have an expression: No one ever quit because they were succeeding. People give up and drop out after a serious setback. It is easy to get discouraged, to feel embarrassed, and to feel alone. I know this from research, but I also know it from personal experience.

I'm not perfect. We've established that. But perhaps what I do pretty well is build my guilty-as-charged moments into my overall plan. Here are two examples of indulgences with happy endings.

## BLOWING IT OUT (THE RIGHT WAY)

One day during the summer of 2009, my first summer on maintenance, I was having a tough day/week/month/lifetime, so I went to a nice little Belgian restaurant a few blocks away from the office. My goal was simple: To eat my way back to an even keel. Right, I was going against most of the advice contained in this book so far.

The waiter announced, "Avoid the fish," but he did have kind words for the roasted pig's head (yikes), fries with a bacon-infused mayonnaise (evil, but tempting), and four-story lamb belly confit (whatever that is). I ordered a cheeseburger, for which the place is known. It rocked. Hard. So did the fries and that mayonnaise. If I am going to throw it all up in the air, I want it to be worth it. No blowing Points values on crummy bad food. Just excellent bad food.

But here's the key to the story: The next day, I resumed making pretty good choices. No harm, no foul.

# RECOVERING FROM A BIG SPILL

In mid-2011, I was at the tail end of a fairly brutal travel schedule. I knew that I had been straying off plan, and I had been studiously avoiding the scale. But at 6 p.m. on a Saturday night, I was fishing something out of the guest room closet, where I keep our Tanita medical scale, and I had the sudden impulse to man up and step on it. Six pounds over goal. Ugh. I went into tailspin mode, grabbing and shaking the fat around my waist and cursing at myself.

Boy, did I suck.

Two observations about this mishap:

**1. What's with avoiding the scale?** There is something dumb and self-destructive about avoiding weigh-ins. I know that I'm slipping, yet somehow denial will make the weight disappear. In the process, I miss the opportunity to quickly self-correct and return to sane choices. Avoiding weigh-ins results in an escalating cycle of not-so-awesome choices followed by further avoidance. This, my friends, equals 6 unnecessary pounds hanging around my waist.

Lesson for me? I remind myself to take advantage of the meetings, which I am already attending for work purposes, and get regular weigh-ins. Lesson for you? Honesty begins with being honest with yourself.

**2. What's with the self-flagellation?** I had been at my goal weight, not moving more than a couple pounds in either direction for well over 2 to 3 years. It was only natural for me to be disappointed and irritated with myself now that I had significantly deviated from this. Fessing up to this publicly, either on my blog or at a Weight Watchers meeting, would be a better way to exorcise the demon—by being honest about the fact that I slipped up. This is the opposite of denial.

In summary: Denial + self-abuse = unhelpful. Honesty + self-belief = good outcomes. There. That feels much better.

# Staying on Maintenance (Without Driving Away Your Friends)

## DON'T BE A BLOWHARD, KNOW-IT-ALL, OR SHOW-OFF

When I was losing my weight, I definitely talked about it in various forums: meetings with staff, family, coworkers, at Weight Watchers meetings, etc. I was part of the crowd that was sharing the struggle. When I went into my maintenance phase, my need to talk about it did not subside. I even started my blog so I could talk to yet more people about it. Some people found this a bit irritating.

From the perspective of people just beginning this process, hearing from people on maintenance can be either incredibly motivating or intensely grating. Why is that? Specifically annoying attitudes among those on maintenance include:

**1. Look at me, dammit! I'm thin!** It's been a great accomplishment for me to lose weight and keep it off, and I'm proud of it. I really like compliments and accolades, because of my inherent shallowness. However, it's kind of sad to ask for compliments (even in a passive-aggressive sort of way).

**2. You should learn from my example!** There are few people more in-your-face than the recently converted. We have a tendency to proclaim our healthy lifestyle at excessive decibel levels. "NO THANK YOU, WAITER, I DO NOT WANT ANY DESSERT." Ex-smokers can be guilty of this as well.

**3. Am I disciplined or what?** I push myself pretty hard on the lifestyle thing, and I don't mind others knowing about it. It would be nice if they would take the time to heap praise upon me and perhaps carry me on their shoulders while running off the field.

**4. Yes, in fact, I am all-knowing.** I possess all useful tips and knowledge about successful weight loss, and it is my right to dominate every conversation to ensure that all others benefit from my vast and unending expertise.

It isn't wrong to feel good about succeeding, but you don't want to do it at the expense of those around you. I need to make it less about me, and more about wanting to help the people I care about. This will help me lower the volume a bit.

# BE A NICE GUEST!

Our founder Jean Nidetch once noted that naturally thin people don't tend to eat all that much food. They usually do not finish what's on their plate. They may eat a bite of dessert, but they will usually stir it up with a fork so it looks like it's been eaten. In other words, they don't make a big deal out of the fact that they don't eat every single thing in front of them. If anything, they try to act like they are big eaters, even though they aren't.

I am starting to think that naturally thin people might be on to something. If I always make a lot of noise about the fact that I'm being careful about what I eat, it's inevitably going to create awkward situations for the people around me. That in turn can make it harder for me to fully live in the real world. This in turn makes it harder to create truly sustainable eating habits.

It's one thing to ask the people who are incredibly close to you, like your family, for their support in helping you stay on program. Most other people do not need to know. Or at least they don't need to know during the act of eating. In fact, I suspect it gets a bit grating for people to listen to others constantly talking about their eating regimen.

Your goal is to navigate real-world situations without having to ask for special help from your host. In addition, you would do well to consider that a friend is not a restaurant proprietor. It's perfectly fine to ask your server to bring dressing on the side or to prepare your food more simply. I'm pretty sure that Emily Post would instruct us that this is not proper etiquette with friends.

Therefore, maybe the alternative is to quietly engage in healthy habits, without verbal accompaniment poured all over it or even on the side.

After all, I'm not on a diet. I'm just living my life.

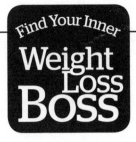

## A future of maintenance can be daunting. Here's how to approach it in the right spirit.

### Stick with it.

If you have had a problem with weight, you will always have to watch what you do. We can manage weight, but it will require a certain amount of effort and diligence. In this context, it might be best to think of a weight problem as a sort of chronic condition. Brushing my teeth is a chore, but it's worth doing to avoid dentures. Putting effort into my nutritional health and fitness is similarly worth it—the alternative is not at all lovely.

### Dance with the one who brought you.

That's an old baseball saying: If it worked to get you to the World Series, stick with it in the World Series. Whatever you are doing to lose your weight must be what you are willing to do forever. Remember: Eating healthy foods is simply what you do now. The same kinds of healthy foods that helped you lose weight are the exact same ones that will help you keep it off. Therefore, choose foods and routines that make you happy and that you can live with.

### There are two sides to the weight loss coin, and they're both good.

We need to live a life where we eat smart and stay active. Two sides, same coin. Heads you win, tails you win bigger.

### Keep fighting.

Weight loss is a battle. Weight maintenance is peace. But peace can allow you to relax your vigilance. So I invent battles as needed. The doctor's visit. The vacation in some warm place where I'll be seen half-naked. The seasonal change of clothes; will they still fit me? Setting short-term goals with implied rewards is a useful tool for giving maintenance a level of urgency.

## Weight Watchers Profile

### "Arming myself—and my kitchen—put me in control again."

Tweak the temptations, seize control of your weight

**Mary Dalton, 53,** *Joliet, IL*
**HEIGHT:** 5 feet 6 inches
**WEIGHT BEFORE:** 226
**WEIGHT AFTER:** 156
Reached her goal in 29 months

### MY STRUGGLE

I first joined Weight Watchers in college and lost 25 pounds. I loved it so much I became a Weight Watchers leader. But when I got married and pregnant with my fourth child, it was like a green light to eat. I thought, "I'm pregnant. I can eat whatever I want." It backfired. The older you become, the more difficult it is to lose weight. I simply couldn't lose the 70 pounds I put on when I was pregnant with my fourth child.

### MY WAKE-UP CALL

I remember seeing the number on the scale: 226 pounds. It was close to what Oprah weighed at one point. To make it worse, as a Weight Watchers leader, I was always aware of how others at the meetings viewed me. I wanted to be a role model—instead, I felt self-conscious.

### MY FOOD

I was a closet eater. I'd slide a candy bar up my sleeve, then hide the wrappers in my coat pocket. I felt guilty, frustrated, out of control. I've changed that. Now, I cook my own meals. My specialty is pasta with chicken-vegetable stir-fry. I chop vegetables and chicken, and throw it over a reasonable portion of pasta. I stock my freezer with chicken, lean ground beef, ham, and salmon. For snacks, I have air-popped popcorn with butter spray. Eating fruit throughout the day—my favorite is grilled pineapple—curbs my cravings for sweets. Arming myself—and my kitchen—with these foods has put me in control again.

### MY FITNESS

I love being outside. So I started my exercise routine with just walking 15 minutes a day. Now I'm up to 1 hour a day and walking 3 to 5 miles. I wanted to add more exercise, so I joined a gym and started circuit weight training. Eventually, I was able to do a 60-minute Spinning class and tried kickboxing! I'm now a personal trainer at my gym and help others achieve their goals.

### MY PAYOFF

Twelve years after I lost the weight, I was diagnosed with breast cancer. But I never thought I couldn't

conquer it. And I knew I didn't have to do it alone. That attitude came from Weight Watchers. It helped prepare me to deal with the tidal wave of emotions: shock, anger, denial and fear, just to name a few. And just like members supported me with my weight loss, they helped me with my cancer. They called, sent cards, and participated in awareness walks. Now I'm 6 months cancer free and am already starting to work out again. I sincerely thank Weight Watchers for allowing me to say, "I am a breast cancer survivor."

# {CHAPTER 10}

# Navigating Trouble Spots—

## Don't Let the "Real World" Keep You Down

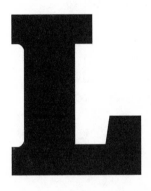**IFE GETS IN THE WAY SOMETIMES.** We don't have the luxury of living in a world of perfect circumstances and predictable events. We are expected to live in harmony with others, not bend them to the needs of our newfound healthier lifestyle. We want to believe that we can live a full life that does not require us to exist in a plastic bubble.

The problem with our messy reality is that it can cause us to quit our efforts to clean up our lives. We tumble from lunch with a client into a weeknight dinner with friends followed by a weekend spent shepherding out-of-town visitors around our favorite watering holes and eating establishments. Which leads right into a week of business travel. Why not throw in a holiday replete with piles of candy or comfort foods? Then we escape from all that with a family vacation, where our weekly routines go right out the cabana window.

During hectic times, we allow a guilt-free 10-pound gain between Thanksgiving and Christmas. We tell ourselves that we've worked hard, that we deserve a great holi-month, a celebration that is 31 times better than a holi-day. We cut loose on a lifestyle sabbatical that we promise will last only 4 weeks—make it 6—before we return to our better habits.

But that moment of return is precisely when many of us quit for good. After wobbling for weeks, we fly spectacularly off the rails and hold ourselves in bitter contempt for our weaknesses. I know this because the we I'm talking about is actually me. When I'm in a normal routine at home, my healthiest habits are in place. Home is the place for predictable and comfortable routines. I really don't have to make a lot of decisions—and we know where those decisions get you. Free me from my routines, though, and I might as well be a wild animal prowling the junk-food jungle for food.

Over the past 10 years, I've learned to troubleshoot many eating scenarios. But I still have serious weak points. Here's how I try to shore them up by relying on years of advice, tips, and lore that I've learned in meetings, taught to me by both leaders and members.

# Restaurants:
# Eating Out, Pigging Out (Same Thing)

One of my all-time favorite B-movie slasher flicks is a gem from the early '80s called *Motel Hell*. In it, a couple of innocent kids find themselves with a malfunctioning car in a small southern rural outpost. They check in to a creepy motel whose proprietors pride themselves on their tasty dried meats. Right: They serve their customers well. Actually, well done. Lesson: Restaurant food is packed with surprises. You never know what (or who) might be in your meal. If you're trying to eat healthy food, you've got to be discriminating.

- **Just because the menu says chicken or fish doesn't make it a good choice.** Even after I joined Weight Watchers, I often found that I was guessing wrong when I tried to choose the healthier option.

- **Fast food joints aren't the only ones who are supersizing.** Restaurants increasingly seek a competitive advantage by giving their patrons "good value" in the form of silly amounts of food. A seemingly safe trip to the local tavern can easily lead to a 1,500-calorie food-and-drink fiasco.

- **On any restaurant menu, about 85 percent of the food is meant for special occasions.** Beer in buckets. Appetizers in baskets. Slab steaks. Five-spoon desserts. But since Americans now spend almost half of their food dollars away from home, this holiday food approach becomes downright dangerous. Of course I want the 12-ounce steak with grilled onions, bacon, and blue cheese on top. I am human, after all. We naturally crave reward foods, not the daily healthy stuff. But we have to find our way to the latter if we want to live the lean life.

I eat out a lot. My social life and my work life pass through restaurants. I don't have much choice in the matter, and anyway, I don't want to live as a shut-in. So my only choice is to stay true to my best dietary habits even when I eat out. I make a handshake deal with myself that I will splurge and go for a bad-food meal only when I really need it. The rest of the time, I stay sane. Here's how I do that.

**Research ahead.** Chain restaurants usually post nutritional information online. For the rest, a menu scan in advance—preferably when you're not starving—will help you quickly identify four or five choices that will taste great and keep you within your calorie budget. There's a reason why David Zinczenko's *Eat This, Not That!* series has sold a gazillion copies; it's definitely worth a spot on your bookshelf. Or in the glove box. When I plan my order ahead, I never (hardly ever) have to worry about being derailed by a bout of food lust. If a chain does not post information, it is sending you an important message: Everything is most likely bad for you, with the possible exception of the ice water.

**Say no to bread plates.** Weight Watchers veterans have been minding this one for years. The bread basket and those adorable rosettes of butter can quickly tack on 200 to 400 calories of mindless eating before you even get started. Most servers will be happy to boost their tip by diverting the bread basket. If one does arrive, consider hiding under the table.

**Develop keyword scanning skills.** When I go through a menu now, I look for friendly words and unfriendly words. Friendly ones include grilled, poached, lightly sautéed, and steamed. The unfriendlies include fried, stacked, lard soaked, stuffed, au gratin, smothered, buttery, creamy, and most cutesy southernisms ("po' boy," "mamma's," "hush puppies"). Two of my favorite words—crispy and crunchy— have been subverted, because they're often synonymous with triple deep-fat fried.

**Ask for dressing on the side.** Okay, you knew to do that. But do you actually do it? Really? I should also more routinely ask for sauces to come on the side, lest they end up on my backside.

**Manage your portion.** In our supersize world, an appetizer is often the size of an entrée from a previous era. So order one for your main course. Women seem much more comfortable doing this than men (i.e., me). And yes, it does seem a bit dainty. In that case, be super-romantic and share an entrée with your partner, so you'll each get the half portion that would be just about right. Of course, that won't work for a meal with your boss. In those situations, I try to make it a point to purposely leave about one-third of my food on my plate. It's still hard for me to do, but it happens more often than not.

**Talk a lot.** I'm told that in some cultures, conversation is an integral part of the dining experience—as opposed to my world, in which I vacuum food without taking a breath, let alone uttering a syllable. There was a study of guys that showed that when they ate with their buddies, they consumed 37 percent more calories than when they dined with their significant other. My theory: She asks so many questions, your mouth is busy with activities other than eating. All for the good.

# Holiday Hazards

Our semiannual food binges are tricky because they come with aftereffects. Before the holiday itself, there is a sudden buildup of bad food inventory in the form of cookies, candies, gift baskets, and—in the wake of giant family meals—leftovers, desserts, and hostess gifts. This horrific path of destruction continues far beyond the actual holiday. It's kind of like a hurricane that strikes the coast of Florida, then continues up the East Coast, inflicting damage long after its initial landfall.

Let me pull on my Weather Channel parka and talk about the damage these storms inflict.

## HALLOWEEN

Research just in: Even small packets of candy have calories. And most have fat. A few fun-size facts:

- One measly Reese's cup: 150 calories
- One solitary, sad Hershey's kiss: 50 calories
- One "fun" size bag of M&M's: 100 calories
- One "fun" size bag of Skittles: 100 calories
- One "fun" size Almond Joy: 100 calories
- One of those little tubes of Smarties: 50 calories

All of the above consumed at once: priceless. Okay, technically, 550 calories. Seem like an extreme example? Please. I'm not sure who came up with the moniker "fun" to relate to teeny-tiny calorie bombs, but I would have used the term "deadly." (Do you think a "deadly size" Almond Joy would sell well?)

Three or four pieces of candy per night may not seem like a big deal, but it pretty much is. It amounts to about 400 calories and is roughly equivalent to eating an extra hot dog on a roll each night. For a month. It's no wonder why people, including me, tend to gain weight this time of year.

My strategy: Dip into the trick or treat basket on the actual night. After that, I leave my kids' candy alone. Not that I have much choice—my kids don't approve of theft, so they monitor my compliance.

# THANKSGIVING

This holiday seems to exist so we can gorge ourselves on massive quantities of food, with the secondary benefits of enjoying family, friends, and yet another Detroit Lions game. I know there were Pilgrims involved as well, but who really focuses on this after the age of 9?

Here is how I approached it pre-enlightenment. Before dinner was even served, I would make my way to the huge layout of appetizers in the form of dips and cheeses, and employ my robotic arm from platter to mouth until I was pretty full. I would then proceed to the buffet, and start heaping as much Thanksgiving dinner on my plate as I could possibly fit. Are you a vegetable? I'm sorry, there is no room for you on my special holiday platter. Only starches are allowed in this loading zone. Dessert? Times three. It would be rude not to have a fat wedge of each pie on the sideboard. I leave the table feeling totally bloated and with a hideous case of heartburn, but still make room for football-related snacks, beverages, and the Detroit Lions.

Urp. Thank you.

Aside from my private misdeeds, Thanksgiving has three problem areas from a weight management perspective.

- The meal itself is often a spectacular display of excess. Do you see marshmallow-topped sweet potatoes any other day of the year?

• The weekend turns into a 4-day bender that really does not end until the last piece of pecan pie is eaten, usually by me at 2 a.m. on the following Tuesday.

• Thanksgiving is merely the opening indulgence in the month long bacchanal known as "the holidays."

How do I handle Thanksgiving? Well, I would never track calories for the actual meal. I'm entitled to let go and not be my normal exacting self. That said, I employ a couple of strategies to head off the disasters of holidays past.

**Avoid the appetizer tray.** The Pilgrims didn't nosh on dip, so I'm being historically faithful if I don't either. That said, if there is a shrimp cocktail tray, I will definitely hit that.

**Eat it all (including green things).** For the actual Thanksgiving dinner, I sample everything, including the vegetables. They tend to crowd out that fifth scoop of stuffing, in my experience. Dessert? You bet. One normal slice of the blue ribbon winner of the pie contest suffices. From here, I go home feeling happy and well fed, but not like a goose stuffed for his appointment at the fois gras factory.

**Beware the post–Turkey Day stuffing.** When the big meal is over, you still have 3 days of free time to go. Ordinary life should resume, along with extra amounts of exercise because of all that free time, and no more Lions games. Because, if you're not careful, Thanksgiving weekend can extend indefinitely into . . .

# CHRISTMAS

For many years of my life, the interval from Thanksgiving to New Year's Day was 40 days and nights of dietary debauchery. The Monday following Thanksgiving marked the beginning of shipments of gift baskets from vendors that would litter the cubicles of our offices. Then came holiday parties, Christmas cookies, and general merrymaking. I would careen into Christmas Eve at the end of 12 days of eating constantly. I would then top it all off by going to an all-day football party at a friend's house on New Year's Day. How could I not gain at least 10 pounds after 5 weeks of this nonsense?

The challenge for many of us is to treat this holiday haze like any other time of the year. This does not mean that we have to throw in our lot with Ebenezer Scrooge and kick carolers in the shins. Rather, we should rely on the same tools that work for us during the more rational parts of the year (i.e., tracking calories, stepping on the scale, etc.). I am always amazed, but not surprised, how many people stop going to Weight Watchers meetings or visiting the Web site during this period. It's the time of maximum temptation, so it should also be a time when our servers melt down because of increased, desperate traffic.

Having documented my year-end excesses, I'll share the plan that saves me from them on a semiannual basis. This is the one I wrote for myself two years ago to get through the season's grand finale. Now, when the sleigh bells ring, I'm ready.

- **DAY 1** (December 23): Start with a huge workout. Have a healthy breakfast and lunch. Spend time with the family in the city doing the big Christmas thing (just dodging the Salvation Army bell ringers provides a surprising amount of exercise). Preselect my dinner options from the restaurant menu on the Internet.

- **DAY 2** (Christmas Eve): Keep it together for breakfast and lunch. Have a huge workout. Abandon reason and planning for Christmas Eve dinner at friend's house. Choose not to have remorse.

- **DAY 3** (Christmas Day): No exercise. Rich food. Candy. More candy. No remorse.

- **DAYS 4-5** (Boxing Day and Day after Boxing Day): I've never celebrated Boxing Day before, but why not? Will plan to get workouts in (probably not huge ones) to mitigate some of the damage. Not planning to be perfect this weekend.

- **DAYS 6-8:** Exercise like a maniac. Live like a coldhearted Puritan for all breakfasts and lunches. Keep it sane for dinner. Avoid stealing candy from my children.

- **DAY 9** (New Year's Eve): Big workout again. Keep it sane for breakfast/lunch. Behave poorly New Year's Eve.

- **DAY 10** (New Year's Day): Rub temples gently. Then eyes. Funnel remorse into a big workout. Keep it pretty normal.

- **DAY 11:** Back on plan.

Damage: Eight to 10 meals not on program; roughly 24 meals on program. This translates into about a 27 percent indulgence rate, which seems manageable for a young(ish) man on maintenance. I also had a dietary airbag deployed: Ten days of exercise would minimize the impact of my calorie crashes. Another mitigating factor: I give myself a buffer zone at the end, to work myself back into shape. And through it all, I have firmly in mind that I will spend January working back down to fighting weight.

This leads to one of my golden rules of staying on program: Avoid getting in so deep that you drown rather than swim for your life. We can all see 5 pounds as a pretty manageable amount of damage to reverse. Once that number hits 10 or more, it's dragging you under, and you start believing the naysayers who are cheering your failure because it justifies their own. It's the shadow of Weight Watchers: the Weight Scoffers. Why not avoid joining their lifetime membership of despair and defeatism by focusing more attention on preventing a huge gain in the first place?

# Travel Pitfalls

Each of us has something in our life that sabotages all of our good intentions and efforts. For some, this can be taking care of endlessly hungry kids at home. For others, it can be eating out frequently. For me, it's travel.

I travel constantly. It's pretty rare that I have a month without at least one flight, and in many of them, I'm out of the office more than I'm in it. That means I am ripped out of my routine and forced to deal with an unpredictable world. Much of my travel is overseas, which results in a combination of long flights and jet lag. Sleep deprivation has been show to mess with hunger hormones, which leads to overeating. So on the road, I'm toast.

Once we are in a different environment (a hotel, a different city, etc.), we can often find ourselves saying "Well, this is different and temporary, so I can make different choices and let things go." This is not a good strategy!

My first strategy when I'm someplace else is to eat exactly the same meals that I would eat at home. For breakfast, this means my usual oatmeal/fruit/yogurt combination. I try to continue the same pattern during lunch and dinner.

My second strategy is to book hotels with really good gyms either on the premises or within walking distance. In many cases, the hotel will allow you to buy a day pass for about $10, which to me is a small price to pay to keep myself sane and fit.

The point of this is simple: Honor your routines. If you are able to stick to your regular patterns even when you are far from home base, it's easier to stay on your program. That is the beauty of routines: They do not require decision making. They are automatic.

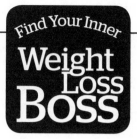

**Life is studded with challenges—the holidays, restaurants, travel. Have a plan. And for heaven's sake, don't throw it all away.**

## It's a holi-day, not a holi-month.

The end of the year isn't a 6-week excuse to binge. Enjoy the big days, but return to sensible eating and exercise plans when you're not literally standing under the mistletoe. Likewise, Halloween is one night at the end of October, not an excuse to eat "fun-size" candy for the month of November.

## Restaurants can be scary.

Americans spend almost half their food dollars at restaurants. That's a problem, because dinner out is a collection of food events you can't control: The chef decides the recipe, the restaurant sets the portion size, and the bartender lowers your inhibitions. It can be a recipe for dietary disaster. So research the menu ahead, make a sensible meal plan, and bring half your dinner home in a doggie bag. Leftovers rule.

## Healthy routines.

Don't leave home without them. We're vulnerable when we travel. Our home habits and safeguards may not seem like they fit in the carry-on luggage, so we often abandon sense when we step on an airplane. Don't. If you work at it, you can replicate your home meal plan, exercise habits, and sense of control no matter where you are. Stick to your routines. They'll see you home safely.

## Weight Watchers Profile

### "Now I do only the things I love."

Food will always be the priority, but fun has its benefits, as well

**Elizabeth Josefsberg, 41,**

*South Orange, NJ*

**HEIGHT:** 5 feet 5 inches
**WEIGHT BEFORE:** 180
**WEIGHT AFTER:** 130
Reached her goal in 2 years

### MY STRUGGLE

I was about 12 years old when my weight issues started. Even then, I was so desperate to lose weight that I'd beg my parents to pay for this diet program for me. I needed to lose about 20 pounds at the time, and I opted for a highly restrictive program that inevitably started my cycle of ups and downs. I would diet for a while, reach my goal weight; then I'd start eating the way I used to and gain it all back. I did that five different times over the course of the next 15 years.

### MY WAKE-UP CALL

By the time I was my heaviest, I had been yo-yo dieting for years. When I was trying to lose weight, I'd eat nothing—maybe 800 or 1,000 calories a day—and I exercised to the extreme. Then, when I wasn't watching my weight, I'd go crazy. One day, while at lunch with my sister-in-law, I noticed she looked great and asked her secret. She'd lost 10 pounds on Weight Watchers. I was curious. I still remember going through the door, thinking I'd be the person to prove them wrong. Once they explained the Points system, I just couldn't believe that anyone could lose weight using it. You have to not eat to lose weight! I thought I knew everything. I decided to give it 1 week, nothing more. So for the next 7 days, I dutifully wrote down my

Points values, stayed in my budget, and I ended up losing 4 pounds! It blew my mind, and I stuck with it.

## MY FOOD

Astoria, Queens, where I used to live, is famous for its bakeries. There were three on my block alone. If I was having a bad day, I'd exit the train, pop into each bakery, and eat everything I'd bought that night. So much of my eating was like a chemistry experiment—it was fake food, and I was always hungry. Today I feel healthier and more energized, and I've worked processed food out of my diet. Now my typical breakfast is berries with Greek yogurt, with a little bit of granola or cereal. I love chicken in the slow cooker over bulgur, spinach, and goat cheese. Travel is a part of my work, so I plan for it. I'll pack a bag with oatmeal packets, 100-calorie almond packs, popcorn, fruit, Babybel cheese, and a treat, so I have options in case of a layover.

## MY FITNESS

The Points system taught me that I can't use exercise as an eraser, and it stopped me from being so extreme. Now I do only the things I love—Spinning one day, running the next, swimming with my kids, tennis. Last year, I was even certified as a personal trainer. I recently did a marathon, and I've done a couple of mud runs. It's finally a joy to be active. I look forward to it every day.

## MY PAYOFF

I feel like the most changed person in the world. I've learned that when you start to take care of yourself, everything improves. My finances are in order, my house is in order, my family relationships are great. Before, I would distract myself by eating so I never really felt my feelings. I feel more assertive now; I'm more aware of who I am, what I want, and what I don't want. I'm stronger.

# {CHAPTER 11}

# Men and Weight Loss—

## Losing Weight Is Not Losing Manhood

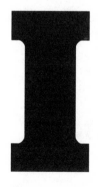**AM A GUY,** and I talk about weight loss in a vaguely personal way. That makes me a somewhat unusual animal. Show me a guy talking about dieting and I will show you someone who is highly likely to be in a twisted state of discomfort.

It's a topic that men have been willing to discuss since, well . . . never. We guys do not have the benefit (or curse) of having spent the last five decades obsessing about weight, except when our significant others droned on about it.

But I wonder if men and women are all that different in the ways they think about weight loss. They may use different words. For example, men "get fit" while women "diet." Yet, are the underlying issues as different as we think, or are men simply less evolved on this topic?

# Men and Denial

To put it all in perspective: Men in this country are at least as likely to be overweight or obese as women, yet we are half as likely to do anything about it. Not good, guys. Maybe it's a motivation problem. For years, women have been browbeaten by themselves, their friends, their parents, the fashion industry, magazines, TV, and their boyfriends and husbands to look a particular way. Yet men have largely gotten a free pass on dealing with weight for vanity's sake—though, as I will discuss later, this is starting to change.

A lot of guys live in a state of denial about the impact of weight on health. And yet, I know any number of guys (me, for one) who get their oversize boxers in a twist when they discover that they are either overweight or obese, according to their BMI number. Their first reaction is to tie it in with global warming: They call it an irritating fantasy dreamed up by science people to make the rest of us as miserable as they are. Don't these white coats know the natural law that men are supposed to be bigger than women?

Yet, if we simply look at the health risk factors associated with BMI, it's pretty clear that men start to run into statistical trouble when their BMI nudges past 25. It's hard for a lot of guys to face the trouble that lurks beyond that number.

# Cultural Norms Gone Horribly Awry

Why do so many men consume massive quantities of food and then beat their chests in victory? What hereditary forces doom guys to a life of overabundance and type 2 diabetes? I blame all of my own behavioral failings on hidden societal pressures dating back to ancient Mesopotamia. Really, if the Assyrians had been a little more thoughtful, they would have established a culture of mindful eating, which then would have spread over Greece, Rome, and ultimately the parts of Europe that were snacking on bone marrow at the time.

Men in these societies were perfectly happy to eat until they had to vomit. The Romans were good at this. Lord knows the Mongols who sacked them were big feasters. To cook "leg of mutton," they burned down the village surrounding a tasty-looking sheep. From that point, the next stop was the Super Bowl. It's totally not my fault.

Think I'm making up this stuff about manly eating? Witness yet another fascinating experiment by Brian Wansink, head trickster over at the Cornell school of test-subject deception. In one experiment, he and his team found that women ate less popcorn when they paid attention to how much they were eating. Makes sense, right? But in the same study, when guys paid attention to how much they were eating, they ate more.

A second experiment was even more telling. Dr. Wansink and his merry pranksters wrote two scripts of a guy on a date, and assigned 140 college men and 140 college women to read one of the two versions aloud. Cue the scary music: Something bad is about to happen. In one version, the guy in the story ate a couple of handfuls of popcorn. In the other, he ate almost all of his popcorn.

After the dramatic performances were over, they conducted the survey. The results:

- **THE COLLEGE MEN** rated the guy who ate almost all of his popcorn as stronger, more aggressive, and more masculine than the guy who picked at a few kernels. In fact, when asked how much they thought he could bench-press, guys predicted the full-box guy could bench-press an average of 21 pounds more. And popcorn was not even a central point of the story!

- **THE COLLEGE WOMEN** were a little more sensible. They didn't rate either popcorn eater as stronger or more masculine. In other words, she's not watching how much you eat, guys, so you can drop the freaking tub!

Actually, I have another theory about what's at work here. We've all heard that women exercise and dress nicely to impress one another, not the men in their lives. Is it possible that we men are inclined to clean our plates in an effort to impress each other? Is this the food version of antler wars?

Since throwing myself into this healthy life/Weight Watchers thing, I have taken lots of grief from my buddies about what I eat. They all tell me—repeatedly, and in creative ways—that I eat like a girl. I have even accused myself of eating like a girl, because in fact I do kind of eat like a girl. So what do I mean by "eat like a girl"?

Consider these cultural icons that define manly eating (since the time of the Mesopotamians):

- **Fred Flintstone:** I'll need to ask our nutritionists to calculate the Points value of Brontosaurus ribs. Anything large enough to tip your car over can't be a proper portion.

- **Henry VIII:** A big eater and proud of it. Lots of wives, which implies another big appetite.

- **Dagwood Bumstead:** Which reminds me, is it lunchtime yet?

- **Bluto Blutarsky from *Animal House*:** Food fight!

- **The Mad Men:** Always eating steak and slurping cocktails, yet they never gain weight. Only on TV.

Do these raging role models matter? And what about the societal expectations they represent? In fact, I do feel self-conscious when I'm dining with a bunch of dudes and I order a lightly prepared fish; they metaphorically kill, skin, and eat large animals while blood drips down their chins. If there is anyone who shouldn't feel strange about eating carefully, it's me! So if I feel the pressure, how do other guys deal with unstated (or stated) peer pressure to chow down and beef up?

But I'm noticing subtle shifts. These days, if I order first at dinner (or early in the lineup), the guys who order after me often choose fish and lighter dishes, too. It's as if I give them license, by my example, to take their foot off the fat-accelerator pedal. I can almost hear their pleas that I take them to a cruelty-free juice bar.

And you know what? We should go to that juice bar every now and then, when we're not eating hamburgers, grazing at salad bars, and sipping soup. Balance is everything, and that includes a balance between "male" diets and "female" diets. In fact, we are all better off if we eat fruits, vegetables, lean meats/proteins, whole grains, and low-fat/fat-free dairy. We share an interest in sane portions and the

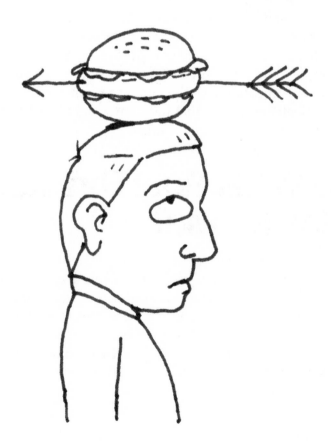

active lives that help us regulate our (predictable) insane moments.

These dietary guidelines aren't just for women so they can help their men get a clue. They're for all of us.

For ages, it seems, women have been dealing with all the issues of body image, which have a big impact on how they think about weight and weight loss. Much has been written about this in too many places to count. That said, I would definitely support the school of thought that the media does no favors with its ritual practice of glamorizing an unattainable or unhealthy body image. If rock-hard abs in a bikini or a size-2 dress is the only definition of weight loss success, we are all doomed to a life of abject misery. We deserve much better than that.

So, what about men and body image?

Let's kick it off with a fun fact. According to Gallup polling, 33 percent of people who are trying to lose weight are doing it for looks, 33 percent are doing it for health, and 33 percent are doing it for both. Suffice it to say, vanity plays a big part in the mix. According to Gallup, men are somewhat more likely to cite health as a driver behind their weight loss, but not nearly as much as you might think.

# So What Role Did Vanity Play for Me?

My official reasons for addressing my weight issue were health concerns such as high blood pressure, high cholesterol, etc. But I knew that something was wrong. I had to see myself in the shower and in the mirror, without the benefit of the camouflaging outfits that filled my closet. That cruel thing that women do when they perform a body critique in the mirror? I did that, too. It's a crummy way to start the morning.

So, if it made me feel bad, why? First, the obvious answer. It's not a great look. I guess that makes me shallow, but honesty is useful here. No matter how hard I tried to suck it in, my layers of flab were the inescapable and not awesome-looking truth. Second, being out of shape wasn't a great statement about me as a person. It was evidence of a lack of discipline and maybe a little laziness. I was embarrassed by the state of affairs.

When I got my offer from Weight Watchers in 2000, I described it to friends as an awesome career opportunity, but I also was secretly looking forward to a possible fix for a hidden (semihidden, anyway) and vexing issue. I wanted Weight Watchers to make me look good naked.

TMI? My apologies. But vanity is a useful secret X factor for lots of people. Maybe you want to look better naked, too? Your secret is safe with me.

# Men, Body Image, and the Media

About a year ago, I saw an article about male mannequins in an issue of *New York* magazine. A British company called Rootstein created its first mannequin in 1956 in London. What has made a bit of a stir recently has been the launch of a new line of male mannequins called Hommes Nouveau. They are crazy skinny. How skinny? A brief history of Rootstein mannequin sizes makes the madness clear.

- **1967** 42-inch chest, 33-inch waist

- **1983** 41-inch chest, 31-inch waist

- **1994** 38-inch chest, 28-inch waist

- **2010** 35-inch chest, 27-inch waist

Really? A 27-inch waist for a guy? A designer from Rootstein said that they use teenage boys as models for the new series of plastic men. Sorry, ladies—they do the same for (to) women!

Now let's pay a visit to the real world, shall we? The CDC's handy National Health and Nutrition Examination Survey has distribution data for male waist circumferences. Here are a few fun facts.

- **1988-94** Average adult male waist size: 37.5 inches

- **1999-2000** Average adult male waist size: 38.9 inches

- **1988-94** Average adult female waist size: 34.9 inches

- **1999-2000** Average adult female waist size: 36.3 inches

A few more interesting stats about that 1999–2000 survey:

- Adult men with a 27-inch waist: about 1 percent
- Adult men with a 33-inch waist (1967 standard): 15 percent
- Women ages 20–29 with a waist size of 27 inches or below: less than 10 percent

You can't look at the male end of the magazine rack without seeing an unending display of six-pack abs. And skinny jeans play a big role in male fashion these days, just as they do in women's attire. There is clearly a disconnect between the ideal male figure you see in a store window and the adult male figure looking in there from the street. It's not hard to imagine how this makes life more difficult for the average guy dealing with a weight issue.

So what about me? Do I look at emaciated male mannequins and beat myself up? Truth be told, I don't really pay attention to mannequins. But I do hold myself to an unreasonable standard, and I tend to be too critical of my swimsuit-wearing self. Am I influenced by the media in this way? I probably am. I probably get more of it from what I see in the movies, and the whole Jersey Shore thing bums me out. We can't all look like The Situation.

I don't even want to. But I do think about it. Which is really pretty sad given that I have been able to shrink my waist from 38 inches to 34 inches. I should be thrilled. And I am, at least until I turn on the TV or step into a news-stand. Unrealistic body images can be unhealthy, unhelpful, and frankly dangerous.

# IS THERE ANYTHING GOOD TO SAY ABOUT MALE VANITY?

I've heard lots of women talk effusively about how, after they lost their extra weight, they had the wonderful opportunity to shop in the "regular" section of women's clothing stores. They talk about being able to show off their arms and legs. They talk about buying pretty clothes, rather than camouflaging ones. They talk about the joy of buying a completely new wardrobe and then using it as a way of motivating themselves not to regain the weight.

What is the equivalent technique for men? Here goes:

I like to buy clothes that make me look thin or fit.

These are the fashion (or style-free) choices that I used to make when I was heavier: anything baggy, loose fitting, or "relaxed fit." Staples included pleated khakis and baggy jeans. I used to wear pretty big, billowing suits and heavy sweaters, the fashion equivalent of sporting a refrigerator box. Because my clothes were big and baggy, I rationalized, wasn't it possible that a skinny guy was on the inside?

As I lost weight, I feared wardrobe malfunctions, but

I enjoyed creating new belt notches to fight them. I started to squeeze up and fold over more and more of the waist on my pants. By the time I reached goal weight, I looked a little like Tom Hanks in *Big*, when he reverted to being a little kid stuck in a large suit.

On an emotional level, this transformation rocked the house. It is hard to express how happy I was when I fit comfortably into 34-inch-waist pants, after years of squeezing into 38s. It was a party in my mind the first time the salesguy at my favorite men's fashion emporium directed me toward styles suitable for, as he put it, "trim men." Hey, that's me! It was shameless salesmanship on his part, and I completely fell for it. He could have sold me anything that day and probably did.

I have now completely replaced my wardrobe, head to toe, and enjoyed every minute of it. For a fat guy, shopping is about deceit and covering up. As a trim guy, I'm showing off. It doesn't feel good to face that fact, but it does feel good to have the body that supports my new vanity.

What does all of this have to do with maintaining my weight? Everything! All of my stuff fits me well now, but a 10-pound weight gain would make me look like a stuffed sausage. Now that Dave is something of a dandy, outfitting him in a bratwurst costume is just not acceptable.

# From Mars and Venus for Real?

Ask a guy with a weight problem if he is an emotional eater, and 9 times out of 10 he will throw a rock at you. But he'll throw it with emotion, and then maybe go have a snack, to feel better. The conventional wisdom is that women eat for lots of reasons that have nothing to do with being hungry, but men eat only when they are hungry. It's just that they are hungry all the time. Because they are men. Make sense?

I'm not so sure.

For those who have never seen one, a focus group is a mainstay of market research that infinite numbers of companies use to gather infinite numbers of opinions on infinite numbers of topics. I've been to a million over my 10 years at Weight Watchers. The most memorable and fascinating ones are when we call in men to talk about weight loss.

Usually, the discussion starts off with a lot of predictable chest thumping and joking, along with proclamations such as "I've got too much pillow in the middle, but it's okay because I'm just gonna start hitting the gym" and "What does it matter if I'm heavy? I'm married!" or "I don't eat because I'm sad. That's for chicks."

What was interesting about the focus groups is how the conversation would change over the course of 60 to 90 minutes. By the end of the sessions, there was a lot of talk about the emotions that accompany those extra pounds and how the extra weight makes guys feel about themselves. These guys usually kept it together, and there was no weeping, but the conversation got pretty personal and very real. The laughter stopped.

So ask me the question. Am I an emotional eater?

Before I answer, let me first provide an honest and important caveat. You can't spend as much time talking about weight issues as I do without developing sympathetic cramping. I'm a much more sensitive dude than I used to be, and, arguably, some of my inherent manliness has been diluted from inhaling estrogen all day, every day, for a decade.

Do I emotionally eat?

Channeling my inner Colonel Nathan R. Jessup, from *A Few Good Men* ... Think of me in the Jack Nicholson role, lecturing the young pup lieutenant, who has a few things to learn.

**COL. DAVE:** You want the truth?

**LT. KAFFEE:** I think I'm entitled.

**COL. DAVE:** You want the truth?

**LT. KAFFEE:** I want the truth!

**COL. DAVE:** Son, we live in a world of cheeseburgers, breakfast burritos, stuffed pizza, and cheese fries. I have my stoic face and crazy disciplined exercise routines to guard against it. Who's going to protect me? You? I have a greater personal responsibility to maintaining my balanced healthy lifestyle than you can possibly imagine. You weep for the fast-food companies, and you curse my disciplined persona. You have that luxury. You have the luxury of not knowing what I know. My failure to finish my dessert last night, while tragic, possibly saved my life. And my established healthy routines, while grotesque and incomprehensible to you, save my life. You don't want the truth because deep down, in places you don't talk about at parties, you want me on that healthy lifestyle. You need me on that healthy lifestyle. I use phrases like "Points Tracker," "Activity Points," "energy density," and "foods with beneficial satiety characteristics." You use them as a punch line. I have neither the time nor the inclination to explain myself to a man who rises and sleeps under the blanket of balanced nutrition that I provide, and then questions the manner in which I provide it. I would rather you just said thank you and went on your way. Otherwise, pick up a Weight Watchers iPhone application and start tracking your snacks. Either way, I don't give a damn what you think you are entitled to.

**LT. KAFFEE:** Do you emotionally eat?

**COL. DAVE:** I handle my feelings the best way—

**LT. KAFFEE:** Do you emotionally eat?

**COL. DAVE:** You're goddamn right I do!

End of hallucination. It's true. I eat for a million reasons that have nothing to do with physical hunger. So what are my emotional trigger points?

• **Boredom:** This is a big one for me. I don't eat much when I'm in the midst of a flurry of activity, running from meeting to meeting or running errand after errand. However, when the air grows still around me, I become ravenous.

• **Stress:** When the weight of the world is on my shoulders and the fates are conspiring against me, I self-medicate with food. I tell myself that I deserve this bit of tasty (nasty) food because life isn't fair. Putting something gross into my system will surely make me feel better. And it does . . . for 3 to 4 minutes.

• **Reward:** This is a BIG yes. I have done great things this week! I deserve a giant reward, preferably with chocolate chips and frozen cookie dough stirred into it.

• **I want to be happy:** Like most people, I've convinced myself that eating can create a state of prolonged joy. It does—if you call a few minutes "prolonged."

• **I want something to look forward to:** I always look forward to my next meal. I like to think that it's because I will get a break or because I will see my family. But it's really because I will see the bottom of my clean plate.

What good is this kind of self-examination?

Knowing your trigger points can be critical to addressing unhealthy habits. Knowing that you are eating for a reason other than being hungry creates the possibility of using cognitive behavioral tools. For example, to fight boredom eating, you just need to replace jaw movement with some other activity. It's incredibly hard to stop a nervous habit unless you replace it with something else.

When I suspect an emotional pig-out, I employ three steps to stop it.

• Identify the emotional trigger that leads to eating.

• Know the warning signs that precede the impulse to eat.

• Have some sort of replacement activity in the wings to take the place of eating.

This might be one way that being a guy can help. Many guys are uncomfortable with introspection, but they pride themselves in being men of action. They like to take steps, follow the instructions, figure it out. And if any of those things can replace that faraway stare when standing in front of an open fridge, a guy can head off weight gain he didn't even know was coming.

If a guy is not willing to admit that he's an emotional eater, he will be doomed to repeat his emotional eating. Men don't get a pass from knowing themselves.

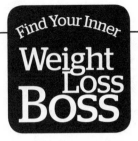

# Guys are just as likely as women to be overweight and half as likely to do something about it. Until now.

## Drop the denial.

Guys make all kinds of arguments: We're supposed to be heavier than women. It's not fat, it's muscle. She likes me this way. Hey, football players are huge, and nobody gives them a hard time.

But here's the fact: Once your BMI nudges past 25, health risks accelerate. If you really aren't buying the BMI argument, then check your waist size: 38 inches or greater is a good indication that it's time to cease the denial.

## Use vanity for motivation—just don't go crazy.

I confess: I like the way I look when I'm skinny and athletic. I also confess that deep down, I really didn't love how I looked overweight, and I really don't much like my before pictures. It's a little sad that I've fallen into the trap of pretty clothes, but frankly they keep me motivated to keep the weight off. Incentives matter.

## Yes, guys are emotional eaters, too.

I'm a focus group of one, so I know. I eat when I'm bored, when I'm anxious, when I'm fidgety, when I need a distraction. Sound familiar? Plan for each of those contingencies and have a strategy to see you through without your eating half a pizza.

## I have a secret for you.

Men can lose weight pretty easily when we put our minds to it. I ate like such an idiot that it was fairly easy for me to drop the pounds. Some women will even tell you (with great and understandable irritation) that it's easier for you to lose weight. Use the early confidence of early weight loss to keep you motivated. Set challenges for yourself and consider using some sort of nonviolent competition with other guys to keep you in the game.

## Weight Watchers Profile

### "I don't feel like I'm on a diet because I'm never hungry."

Lose the weight for your family or someone you love—but do it for your health

### Charles Barkley, 49

**HEIGHT:** 6 feet, 6 inches
**WEIGHT LOSS:** 43 pounds, as of February 2012
**GOAL:** To keep losing!

#### MY STRUGGLE

I know it sounds crazy, but I know more about how to eat healthy now than I did when I was a professional athlete. I played in the NBA for 16 years and I ate anything that I wanted to because my metabolism was through the roof. I had 8.9 percent body fat and I felt like I was a stud. And then I retired and soon found myself in a select category of men, this incredible number of ex-jocks who stopped playing, carried on eating the same food, and got fat.

#### MY WAKE-UP CALL

I'm from Alabama and we're the fattest state: number one in diabetes, stroke, and hypertension. I could see that I'd gotten fat and that among my friends and family I wasn't alone. But for all that, I hadn't had a physical pretty much since I retired, and I was starting to wonder how much I weighed. When I went to my doctor and got on the scale, I thought there was something wrong with it. I was shocked to see that I had gained 100 pounds. My doctor was straight with me. He said, "You're going to drop dead or you're going to have a stroke." The last thing I wanted to do was be an old, fat guy taking a bunch of pills.

#### MY FOOD

I'm still eating the food I love. I mean, everybody likes fried chicken, pizza, and wings, and one of the cool things about Weight Watchers is you can still have them. Should you have five slices of pizza? No. Can you eat wings all day? No. But I still love my fried chicken; I just don't order it every time I eat out, which is a lot. And if there's something that comes with the dish that I don't think is worth the calories, I just ask them to leave it off. I'm much better about eating good stuff all through the day, too. I eat breakfast now, which is new for me. And at night, when I'm at the TNT studios, I get hungry, so I take in my popcorn, my jerky, and my packs of pickles and olives, instead of getting into the barbecue chips. I've found all these new things I like—I make turkey quesadillas, barbecue chicken sandwiches—still real food but lighter than before. But I don't feel like I'm on a diet because I'm never hungry.

## MY FITNESS

When you play sports for as long as I did, everything on your body hurts all the time. Your knees are shot, your back is shot, and the last thing you want to do is go and lift weights and get on a treadmill and elliptical. But even losing the first 20

pounds, I noticed that things got better. I love working out on the elliptical because it's easy on your joints and you can read while you're doing it. I do Crossfit, too—I wouldn't say I love it, but it's just a terrific workout, flipping those big tires around. I have so much more energy now, and it's really exciting to me to see the definition in my muscles coming back.

## MY PAYOFF

I love it when people come up to talk to me about being on Weight Watchers. It seems everyone's got a story about it—they've tried it, or their mom or their wife has. I really hope that I'm going to get more men talking to me about it. I've got a message for these guys: There is no shame in men going to Weight Watchers. I tell people, we don't even need scales. If you want to know if you're fat or not, just stand in the mirror naked—the mirror never lies to you. At some point, you have to address the fact of your weight. Do it for your wife, your girlfriend, your kids. But most of all, do it for your health. The bottom line for me is, I'm getting my sexy back.

# {CHAPTER 12}

# Nobody Eats Alone—

## It Takes a Village to Lose a Pound

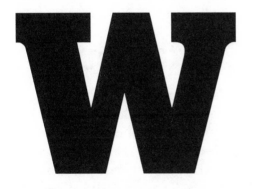**HEN WE'RE THINK-
ING ABOUT LOSING
WEIGHT,** we are not
thinking about the
person sitting next to
us. Our weight prob-
lem feels like it's ours
alone. On some level,
that may be true, but
consider the fact
that 70 percent of the population is classified as clinically
overweight or obese. We clearly aren't alone in our struggles.
When I think I'm having crazy thoughts about my own weight
struggles, all I have to do is look around, and I will see four
or five other people thinking roughly the same set of crazy
thoughts, as reflected in their even crazier behaviors.

The fact that we are not alone with our weight struggles
creates a host of challenges for our society. But there are
opportunities and challenges for each of us individually. It's
not hard to find support or a sympathetic ear. But if we're all
struggling with weight, does obesity become the new normal?
Alternatively, can we use the fact that we struggle with the
same issue as the galvanizing force to beat the obesity epidemic back?

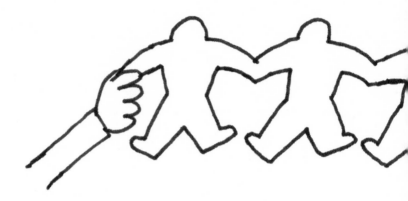

# Is Obesity Contagious?

One of the big head-scratchers for researchers is: To what degree are our lifestyle choices influenced by the choices of people around us? In 2007, two researchers, Nicholas Christakis, MD, PhD, and James Fowler, PhD, did a large-scale analysis to attempt to answer this question. Their results were published in the *New England Journal of Medicine*. They used a huge heap of epidemiological data from the Framingham Heart Study, which allowed them to observe local social networks over a period of more than 50 years. What they found was fascinating.

> • If you have a sibling who is obese, your likelihood of becoming obese increases by 40 percent. This jumps to 67 percent between sisters.
>
> • If your spouse becomes obese, your likelihood of becoming obese increases by 37 percent.
>
> • Most interestingly, if a good friend becomes obese, you have a 57 percent greater chance of becoming obese. If you and your obese friend describe your relationship as "mutually close," your likelihood of becoming obese increases by 171 percent.

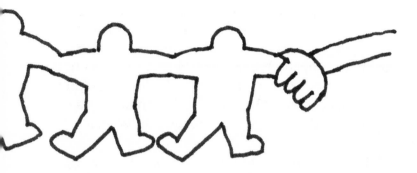

All of this was done while controlling for related factors, such as age and income. Amazingly, the risk of becoming more obese remained high even if you and your friend were geographically separated.

So should we dump all of our friends who are struggling with weight? Should we file for divorce when our spouses gain a few pounds? Obviously not. However, it can come in handy to know that our behaviors are influenced by the people closest to us. There's an upside here: The study's authors also suggest that, if our friends and/or spouse loses weight, we could improve our own odds of losing weight as well.

This makes intuitive sense to me. If I'm spending all of my time with guys who drink a lot of beer, I'm more likely to drink a lot of beer. (Exhibit A: Dave Kirchhoff's idiot college years.) If said friends take jobs and marry and slow down, I'm more likely to do the same. Similarly, if my friends are ordering in a healthy way in a restaurant, I'm more likely to do the same.

Perhaps most important, if as a family we are all trying to live healthfully, our odds can only improve. Yet, the opposite is equally as true. My wife and I have both been marching toward the same set of better food and exercise habits as the years have gone by. I can only imagine how difficult it must be for a husband and wife who are heading in opposite directions.

This gets to the bigger point: It is a lot easier to change your lifestyle as a member of a team than acting on your own. I have seen so many spouses succeed going through this process together. Lots of co-workers have been able to keep one another headed in the right direction, as well. It's easier for us to agree on a lunch spot if we're all looking for the same kind of menu. That's probably why workplace meetings are one of the fastest growing parts of Weight Watchers.

If you're looking for weight loss support from your family, workmates, or social circle, here are a few very basic but important suggestions.

- When you seek a healthier lifestyle, involve your family or at least secure their support.

- Launch your quest with a friend or a group of friends, and keep each other strong.

- If friends and family aren't an option, seek out some other weight control community. The power of mutual support is the entire reason Weight Watchers exists. I know it works.

# Is There a Relationship Between Obesity and Income?

We've seen that there's a relationship between our social circles and the circumference of our waists. Does the content of our wallets play a role, too? From a broad perspective, obesity is—pardon the pun—a mass issue. There are 1.6 billion adults around the world who are overweight and another 400 million who are obese (with a BMI greater than 30). The World Health Organization is forecasting this number to increase to 2.3 billion overweight and more than 700 million obese by 2015. This would suggest that obesity cuts a wide demographic swath.

However, this does not address whether the obesity epidemic has invaded the most wealthy enclaves in America. I don't have statistics on this, but I cannot help but make observations about the town where I live.

My town in Fairfield County, Connecticut, is part of what is historically known as the Gold Coast. This stretch of towns along Long Island Sound (Greenwich, Stamford, Darien, Westport, etc.) is filled with people who commute to well-paying jobs in NYC. I live in a place where affluence and abundance is the norm.

Living in my town is fascinating, particularly as it relates to my job at Weight Watchers. Why? Most people who live here are blond (real or otherwise). They dress well (depending on how one feels about appliqué-whale pants), and they drive nice cars. I'm always struck by the observation my parents made when they first visited me here 10 years ago: They asked, "Where are the heavy people?"

In this town, living in the 1 percent refers to body fat.

It is telling that the original version of *The Stepford Wives* was filmed in a Fairfield County town. Maybe all of the heavy people in my town were replaced by robots? More likely, I would attribute the thinness of my town to the metaphorical lesson from the movie: Peer pressure plays a massive role in how we live. In my curious town, it's just expected that one be thin.

Consider the suggestion in the previous section that obesity might be contagious. As I look around my town, it seems the opposite is also true. If all your friends are skinny, you want to be skinny, too. If you are a skinny female and live in an affluent town, you want to be able to rock a Chanel dress because your friend is swanning about in a Lilly Pulitzer (it's a preppy town, after all). Short of calling the cops, this is how affluent people maintain a sense of order in their community.

I'm not judging this kind of motivation. I'm merely making an observation. From my point of view, health and well-being have always been by far the biggest reasons to move toward a healthy lifestyle. They get me motivated to come to work each day. Yet, vanity and social acceptance have played a role (for better or worse) when it comes to weight management for decades.

So what defines the lifestyle of the women in my town? First off, they work out like convicts. They scoff at the "modest" Physical Activity Guidelines for Americans of 150 minutes of moderate activity per week. This crowd does a brisk business in yoga, Pilates, Spinning classes, boot camp death classes, personal training, tennis, etc. They pretty much work out every day, and they push it. They are competitive and intense when it comes to their exercise, and they take a lot of abuse from their Spinning coaches (or maybe that's just me).

From a food perspective, they eat 90 percent "clean"—that is, they shun processed foods and the drive-thru, and subsist on reduced rations of fish, skinless chicken, and salads. They pick at their food and claim to be gorging—"I ate a whole sandwich! I'm so bad!" If they have one high-calorie vice, it's fermented grape juice.

It's easy to make fun of this crowd ("Eat a sandwich!"), but allow me to recharacterize their lifestyles: They exercise a lot, and they watch what they eat. If the entire country exercised a lot and ate clean, we could forgive everybody a few hits on the Chardonnay bottle, with pinkie delicately extended. And I fully recognize that affluent communities have access to the resources they need to help them maintain a healthy lifestyle. Gaining access to healthy choices is much more difficult process for the great percentage of society, and it borders on nearly impossible for the poorer among our population.

# SO HOW DOES WEIGHT GAIN WORK WHEN POVERTY IS A FACTOR?

In late 2010, I became involved with City Harvest (www.city harvest.org), a wonderful organization serving people in New York City. They operate a fleet of 17 refrigerated trucks and three bikes, to collect food from those who have extra and donate it to those who need. Also great: City Harvest specializes in fresh produce collections and donations. I volunteered at one of their Mobile Markets in the Bronx, in the midst of a large section of low-income housing. The morning I volunteered, City Harvest gave out about 19,000 pounds of produce to roughly 500 people, enough to last them for 2 weeks. It was inspiring for me and helpful for everybody who attended.

Still, I'm sad that this neighborhood even needs a Mobile Market. In fact, we couldn't find any fresh produce within a 10-block radius. Among the other privations they face, people in low-income neighborhoods literally do not have access to healthy foods. Nutrition experts have a term for these areas: food deserts. Yes, you can still eat in a food desert, but often, the only kinds of food available are the processed, sugary, added-fat, empty-calorie kind. Worse yet, the United States has become a place where processed food has gotten cheaper while unprocessed food has grown more expensive. Suddenly it's easier and cheaper to fill a hungry stomach with junk than it is to fill it with nutritious food.

This has led to a phenomenon where those without resources are forced to spend their food money on energy-dense, caloric foods with little to no nutritional value. In the process, obesity has thrust itself into places where people have few options and alternatives. Obesity and poverty have become two sides of the same coin. Diabetes and other conditions are on the rise, and kids are paying a lifelong price. It's a deplorable, heartbreaking situation.

## WHAT CAN BE DONE?

For the past three years, Weight Watchers has proudly supported Share Our Strength (www.strength.org), which has the simple but ambitious goal of ending childhood hunger in our country by 2015. There is a crying need. Seventeen million US children faced chronic hunger at some point last year. The organization was founded by brother and sister Billy and Debbie Shore in 1984, and it has already raised $200 million, which they have donated to more than 1,000 organizations.

The Shores and their crew at SOS are convinced that childhood obesity and hunger are related problems with a joint solution: nutrient-dense foods. You've heard me extol the virtues of such foods as well. It interests me that so many people who are watching the influence of food on society find common ground on that. So it was an easy decision to choose Share Our Strength as the beneficiary of all of my royalties from this book. We all may be taking on different battles in this food fight, but ultimately, we're all trying to head in the same direction—for ourselves, for the least fortunate among us, for our country and world.

I believe in my heart that our efforts to improve nutritional access to those most in need can help us focus on looking after our own health. I have no scientific evidence to support this hypothesis, but some beliefs go beyond the need for proof.

# Does "Healthy" Have to Be Expensive?

It is true that the relative price of what we would call the good foods—organic vegetables and fruits, hormone-free meats, nuts and seeds, fresh herbs—have increased in price much more rapidly than heavily processed foods and drive-thru disasters. On a few levels, this is to be expected. First, agricultural subsidies have given us mountains of corn and soybeans, which have in turn provided the cheap raw materials for processed foods. In addition, large food companies—like any major industry—work assiduously to find efficiencies in how they manufacture their products. It is easier to find efficiencies in a plant making crackers and cereal than it is in an apple orchard. I'm not being critical. The food industry is just doing its job: producing a popular product as cheaply as possible. It's up to us to choose what we buy and eat. Better decisions will make for better products.

Does that mean we have to flock to the local Whole Foods and plunk down our whole paychecks for organic, artisanal everything? Personally, I love Whole Foods so much it hurts. Part of the pain is because it's so expensive and out of reach for many, if not most, people. But there are smart people who take exception to the assertion that good food is expensive food, and they like to point out that if you buy a cheap meal, you'll pay more in future health costs than you save right now at the register.

Not long ago, Mark Bittman—author of the modern classic cookbook *How to Cook Everything*—wrote a passionate column for the *New York Times* arguing that this belief is just plain wrong, if you know your way around some basic ingredients. He pointed out that $14 can buy enough roasted chicken, vegetables, and salad to feed four to six. Try spending $14 at a fast-food joint and see if you can do the same.

Bittman has allies at Weight Watchers. First off, you can eat more vegetables and fruit without ever disturbing those neat produce piles at Whole Foods. Frozen vegetables are inexpensive, and because they're picked at the height of ripeness in the field, they retain flavor and nutrition when they're flash frozen. That Jolly Green dude really knows what he's doing, in fact. And beans are an excellent source of protein, yet they cost . . . beans.

In order to eat these healthy, simple, nutritious foods, we have to be willing to cook them. Bittman is a leader in this movement, because his simple recipes usually pull off the triple play of great taste, few ingredients, and fast cook times. But it's not nearly as easy to eat healthfully if you're allergic to the kitchen. Preparing food does take a little effort, but never as much as we think, especially if a pro like Bittman is guiding you. I'm also a fan of Lisa Lillien (aka Hungry Girl), who has a gift for making lower-calorie food preparation easy and fun.

The extra effort is worth it. Changing your life isn't the easiest thing to do, but it is the best thing you can do.

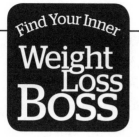

# Each of us focuses on our personal weight issues, but we can be stronger when we join forces—and maybe even help make the world a little better.

## We're all in this together.

Surprising new research shows that we tend to mirror the weight status of those around us. Families grow heavy together, but they can also grow lean together. The same goes for societies. So which will it be? Our individual choices can make a difference to those around us, especially our children.

## Pitch in to help someone else.

There are too many places where making a healthy choice is incredibly difficult. In my backyard in New York City, there are 3 million people who live in so-called food deserts. Schools still have a long way to go to make sure that our kids are getting nutrient-dense foods. Be part of the solution. Get involved in your school's lunch policies. Find an organization that gives people access to healthy food. Share Our Strength and Feeding America are two great places to start. Most important, be a good healthy life role model for your kids or the kids in your life.

## Eating well doesn't have to be expensive.

We're flooded with cheap fast-food options as we drive down the street and inundated with cheap processed foods as we roll down the supermarket aisles. But if you're willing to cook for yourself, a world of inexpensive, healthful options opens up to you. Whole chicken. Fresh vegetables. Milk and cheese. Eggs and more eggs. Turn on the stove and turn off the weight gain.

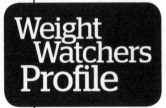

Weight Watchers Profile

## "It's not about what you do. It's about what you choose to do next."

Everybody strays.
The question is: How quickly
can you snap back into line?

**Debbie Hugo, 53,** *Seattle, WA*
**HEIGHT:** 5 feet 3½ inches
**WEIGHT BEFORE:** 167
**WEIGHT AFTER:** 127
Reached her goal in 9 months

### MY STRUGGLE

I don't remember a time I *wasn't* struggling. I never looked like the other girls in school. I was always the chubby one, always the last picked for teams. In seventh grade, my friend and I decided we were going to diet. I had no clue what dieting looked like, except that everyone I ever saw do it didn't enjoy it and ate yogurt! That started my journey toward finding a healthy weight—but too often, that involved taking unhealthy measures that never stuck.

### MY WAKE-UP CALL

For Christmas of '89, my brother received a camcorder. Later that evening, we were watching the playback, and this person walked in front of the camera lens. I was thinking, Who was here that I didn't see? They have a really big butt! And then the person turned around, and it was me. I was so upset—so I had a second piece of pumpkin pie to soothe myself! It took me 3 weeks to actually visit Weight Watchers. When I stepped on the scale, I felt immensely sad. I was going to quit. But then the meeting started, and I thought, Now I'm gonna have to talk really, really loud to tell this lady I'm quitting! So I stayed. I told myself I'd lose 10 pounds and then quit. I did that four separate times, until I'd lost 40 pounds!

### MY FOOD

My biggest change was in awareness—I'm now very conscious of what I put in my body. And I've learned that I don't have to be stuffed every time I'm finished eating. You can only eat what you have, so I strictly buy fruits, vegetables, lean meat, and low-fat dairy. I used to eat potato chips until the sides of my mouth cracked from the salt. I buy baked chips but never the huge bags. I've realized that you can always pick back up if you mess up. It's not about what you do; it's about what you choose to do next.

### MY FITNESS

It wasn't until after I had lost a lot of weight that I felt comfortable in a gym. So while I was losing, I worked out along with a morning exercise TV program every day. Walking was huge for me, and little by little, by empowering myself and starting small, I became more active. The goals kept growing. Last year, I ran a half-marathon. Now I go to the gym two or three times a week, and I walk whenever I can fit it in.

### MY PAYOFF

I'm 53 now, and I'm in better shape than I was at 23. I became a Weight Watchers leader, and several years ago, I had an idea: Members would buy nonperishable food items that weighed as much as they'd lost that week. Then we donated it all to a food bank. Their loss would be somebody else's gain! Helping the community was a huge motivation. Then in 2008, Weight Watchers used my idea as inspiration for the Lose for Good campaign! One little idea has helped countless people across the country. What a great payoff!

# {CHAPTER 13}
# Is It Over Yet?
## Am I Cured?

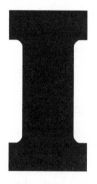AM WRITING THIS FINAL CHAPTER
on a Sunday from a hotel room in San Francisco. Over the next few days, I will attend
a big health care conference where I will be
making the case for the value of proactively
addressing the obesity epidemic as the single
most important way of driving down health
care costs over the long term. I will be representing my company, Weight Watchers, and
the nearly 45,000 people who work tirelessly
trying to make a positive change in people's lives. I hope, as
always, to do right by them, because they deserve my very best.

When I stand up, you can be sure that people will be checking out the guy from Weight Watchers, curious whether he is
at a healthy weight. I am expected to be a role model, and that
is totally fair. I may get the question, as I often do, about what
percentage of people are cured after having gone to Weight
Watchers.

I will make the argument that there is no clear cure for obesity. If you struggle with weight, your temptation to fall back
on favorite decadent habits may never go away. Much of the
research these days suggests that this is true for reasons that
start with your brain and further involve your metabolic and
hormonal systems. Our bodies and minds have evolved over
thousands of years to protect our fat stores.

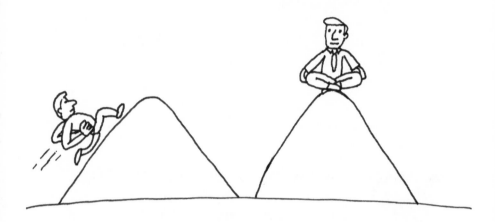

I make this argument because, no matter what you see when you look at me right now, I am not cured.

In this very hotel room, I watched the Giants spank the Atlanta Hawks in the NFL Wildcard game. As I sat there, I grabbed a tube of peanuts and wolfed it down like a starving man, even though I had eaten lunch 30 minutes earlier. After I did this, I went through my normal rounds of self-reproach for being so incredibly lame since I was in town to talk about solutions to the obesity crisis. (Problem #1: Dave.)

Here is my inventory of the list of healthy habits I like and crummy habits I need to keep working on.

### THE GOOD

• In the past 52 weeks, there have maybe been 2 or 3 weeks where I did not get some sort of meaningful exercise for at least 6 of the 8 days of the week.

• In the past 52 weeks, I have probably diverged from my healthy breakfast routine five or seven times, aside from my allowed Saturday-morning cereal-fest indulgence.

• I can almost always make a good choice for lunch or dinner.

• I snack on an apple at 3 p.m. rather than a bag of cookies or chips.

• In public, you will almost always see me being a very upright nutritional citizen.

## THE UGLY

• I still do too much mindless grazing, particularly after dinner and during the day on weekends. I continue to attribute this to a nervous/compulsive habit resulting from not being busy enough during those times.

• I'm not afraid to shake down a minibar in a hotel room (witness today).

• It's a good thing I'm not a pilot, because I always make bad choices on airplanes.

• I still compulsively clean my plate. Once I get in the eating zone, I can't stop until I've eaten all the way to china.

When I write a list like the one above, I feel like I've made pretty good progress. It's been almost 3 years since I reached my goal weight, and I'm still there. Most people would look at me and say that I'm totally in control, reformed, and cured. Yet maintaining all of my progress requires continuing effort. I still track PointsPlus values even though I really don't like doing so—it's just not in my DNA. Yet I do all of this because it's worth the effort.

When I look at the list of what is working, in every case it is because I have established a routine that requires little or no decision making, including exercise. When I look at the list of my struggles, they are also behaviors that tend to operate on autopilot. I'm barely aware of them when they are happening or they somehow feel out of my control.

All of this comes back to the basic premise of this book: The key to making this work for the long term comes from establishing new behaviors and routines that you can live with. It also comes from creating interventions that interrupt the mindless behaviors that bring us down. Your environment is strewn with hazards, so you have to pick a path that helps you avoid them.

But what's going on in my head—is my brain my own worst enemy?

# Will the Real Dave Please Stand Up?

One of the aspects of maintenance that I struggle with the most is the following nightmare thought—that any day, I will receive the following notice:

> Dear Mr. Kirchhoff,
>
> We have reviewed our records, and it has come to our attention that your visa in our beautiful country has expired. You are now in violation of our laws, and you will be deported immediately.
>
> Thanks for the visit!
>
> Sincerely,
> The citizens of Thin-landia

That's right. I am afraid that I will be discovered as an intruder, not a native citizen of the land of thin people. Then I'll have to go back to where I came from, Heavyopolis.

It's strange how we rigidly define ourselves based on how we once were, particularly when it comes to body image. This makes us second-guess ourselves, and it convinces us that we are ultimately doomed to trudge through life as the never-changing version of our former self. We see ourselves as rubber-band people who will inevitably snap back to our former size. There seems to be a biological underpinning for this elastic effect, but I wonder how much of it is in my head. Like a lot of people, I see myself a certain way, and I assume it represents some inherent truth.

Over the past couple of years, I have taken an interest in studying Buddhist philosophy and its intersection with psychology. Light reading, right? Buddhists have spent the last 3,000 years pondering and analyzing why people think what they think, so I find the Buddhist perspective to be fascinating. One concept I have been particularly intrigued by is reification. It refers to a logical fallacy where we ascribe real-world characteristics to airy, insubstantial ideas.

Huh?

What I mean is, I have this tendency to construct an image of myself carved in stone, based on who I think I am. Family, friends, workmates—even complete strangers—slap on labels and identifiers, and I willingly incorporate them into my design. From what I understand, Carl Jung referred to this as the shadow self, a part of the unconscious mind consisting of repressed weaknesses, shortcomings, and instincts.

Buddhists would tell us two things: (1) This so-called self is full of distorted thinking and misconceptions, and (2) clinging to this image ultimately makes us miserable. They say that there is no "self," that we are all interconnected beings suffering from the same basic stresses. They suggest that the only path to happiness is to have compassion for our fellow planetmates and to let go of our fake selves (i.e., shed our self-images).

At this point, you may be thinking: (1) "Dave, thanks for your attempt to compress an incredibly intricate philosophical worldview into a paragraph; (2) "Dave, this makes my head hurt"; (3) "Dave, you are a strange man, and BTW, can I borrow some patchouli oil?"; or (4) "Dave, what does this have to do with my weight?"

I thought you'd never ask. Welcome to my body image self-portrait gallery. It is comprised of three phases of identity.

- **EMACIATED MAN:** Ages 4 to 17 during which time I was disturbingly thin. Ribs countable, girls repelled, weight gain impossible.

- **BIG MAN:** Ages 21 to 34, during which time I gained roughly 70 pounds (at peak) from where I was at age 17. I became a big guy who was doomed to clean his plate of food as well as whatever was left on his neighbor's plate (even if those leftovers were at a different table in the restaurant).

- **TEMPORARILY FIT MAN:** Age 35 to present. I'm nursing my weight loss along by exercising diligently and eating carefully (except on airplanes, in hotel rooms, on Saturdays in the kitchen . . . ). But I remain the "big man" underneath; I assume it is my nature to eat compulsively because that is "who I am."

Here is my point. The Buddhists are right: There is no firmly defined "me." I am a collection of choices that I make each day, and I am constantly evolving, growing, and changing. I am not bound by who I was when I was 7, 17, 21, or 34. I can make choices each day that are different from ones I made 10, 15, or 20 years ago. I can be Calcified Dave, endlessly repeating negative behaviors, or I can be Dave Unbound, with a world full of possibilities and growth.

So as we look to our futures, in some sense we are all immigrants. We all came from someplace else (the past), but our future can be defined by the choices we make going forward.

Citizens of Thinlandia, I have an answer for you: I plan to stick around a while. I am extending my own visa, in fact, and I'm going to apply for permanent residence.

I belong here.

# Going Forward

It took me 12 years to get where I am. It took more than a fair bit of effort. I have had plenty of moments of doubt and disappointment. And yet, the quality of my life has improved immeasurably.

I'm probably in better shape today than I have ever been in my life, and that's because I'm much more likely to make healthy choices than poor choices. I have gone from being on the verge of diabetes and heart disease to acing all of my health metrics. I also look a lot better than I used to, which is going to make me quite the peacock in the old-folks home one day. I took my job at Weight Watchers thinking it would be a great professional opportunity, and it ultimately changed my life in ways that I never would have imagined or thought possible.

I'm still a work in progress, and I always will be. This is true in every aspect of my life, not just my health. Effort is required, but the rewards are bountiful.

# Why *You're* the Weight Loss Boss

It's dangerous to take advice from a flawed man. You could take my counsel with grains of salt, but it might push you over the sodium limit in your diet. There are many who lost their weight more quickly than I did and who make the whole process seem easier. Yet, between my own personal experience and the vantage point of my job, I have learned a lot.

Of course, I lost weight my way. You'll lose it your way. But our separate odysseys are likely to share a few common ideas.

- **Willpower isn't the answer.** If you keep testing yourself in the face of massive temptation, you will almost certainly succumb.

- **Establish healthy habits.** Displace negative behaviors with new, healthy habits and routines that you don't have to think about. Expect that each habit will take 2 to 3 months to become something you do automatically.

- **Control your environment.** If you find yourself mindlessly eating and falling prey to nasty little behaviors, change the environment so that they are no longer possible. Banish your trigger foods and replace them with healthy favorites.

- **Don't live in deprivation.** If you run around hungry all the time, you will eventually gorge yourself. Starvation is not a weight loss strategy. Instead, find foods that keep you feeling full but are also great calorie bargains. When in doubt, bulk it up.

- **Exercise daily.** This one may be hard, but there is no way around it. You need to exercise pretty much every day, and you need to make it a priority. I strongly preach the good book of resistance training to build muscle (which burns calories at rest by boosting metabolism) as well as cardio. There is no way on Earth I would have been able to maintain my weight loss without working out regularly. The biggest challenge has been to find a way to make it a priority in my schedule every day. I'm a pretty busy guy, so if I can do it, you probably can, too. You just need to make it matter to you.

- **Pull on an awesome tool belt.** Whether you do a program like Weight Watchers or something else, equip yourself with a set of tools and resources that will (1) make the process easier, and (2) create accountability and control mechanisms. If I had not been going to meetings and getting weighed each week, I would not have stuck with my goal long enough for my habits to kick in. If I had not tracked what I was eating, particularly in the early days, I would never have learned enough about foods and calories, nor would I have installed mechanisms to force me to choose differently.

- **Don't go it alone.** This is all so much easier when you have a weight loss partner, particularly if you live with him or her.

- **Give yourself a break.** You will most likely fall off the horse at some point. Maybe you'll fall off repeatedly. When you do, you'll have a choice: stay down or get back up.

You know where staying down will leave you. Don't beat yourself up when you do fall down—it happens to all of us. A lot. It doesn't mean you are weak or lacking character. It simply reflects the fact that being healthy is challenging and takes effort.

So there you have it. Losing weight and keeping it off is not easy, yet it is totally doable. The habits and behaviors you develop in the process are more than worth the effort for your health, regardless of what you think you see in the mirror. On some basic level, each of us has a choice: (1) Seek to be healthier, with the nice side benefit of shedding a clothing size or two; or (2) let health fall by the wayside. For me, this long journey has paid me back more times than I could ever hope to count. My only wish is for you to experience all the same and more.

Cheers,

David

# Index

Underscored page references indicate boxed text.
**Boldface** references indicate illustrations.